The ceremonial

International Library of Sociology

Founded by Karl Mannheim

Editor: John Rex, University of Warwick

Arbor Scientiae
Arbor Vitae

A catalogue of the books available in the **International Library of Sociology** and other series of Social Science books published by Routledge & Kegan Paul will be found at the end of this volume.

The ceremonial order of the clinic

Parents, doctors and medical bureaucracies

P. M. Strong

Department of Social and Community Medicine,
University of Oxford

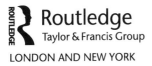

Routledge
Taylor & Francis Group

LONDON AND NEW YORK

First published 1979 by Routledge and Kegan Paul Ltd.

Reissued 2018 by Routledge
2 Park Square, Milton Park, Abingdon, Oxon OX14 4RN
711 Third Avenue, New York, NY 10017, USA

Routledge is an imprint of the Taylor & Francis Group, an informa business

Publisher's Note
The publisher has gone to great lengths to ensure the quality of this reprint but points out that some imperfections in the original copies may be apparent.

Disclaimer
The publisher has made every effort to trace copyright holders and welcomes correspondence from those they have been unable to contact.

A Library of Congress record exists under LC control number: 2001022936

ISBN 13: 978-1-138-73548-4 (hbk)
ISBN 13: 978-1-138-73546-0 (pbk)
ISBN 13: 978-1-315-18650-4 (ebk)

To the memory of my father

Contents

Preface

This is a book about the meetings that doctors have with
parents when a child is sick or needs medical inspection.
(Here and there therapists too will make an appearance.)
It says nothing about the medicine involved in all this
and very little about people's feelings, opinions or perceptions. These things are interesting but they are not
my interest here. My concern is with ceremonies: with
the social form of the occasion and the sorts of identity
tacitly claimed by each party and conferred upon the
other.

One way of seeing it is as a study of 'the doctor-
patient relationship'. Of course parents are not
patients, meetings are not the only part of a relationship, and doctors can meet with patients in a variety of
ways, not just one. All of these qualifications will get
a mention. Nevertheless, the phrase is worth hanging on
to until something more precise - if rather more academic - appears later on.

Research always takes place somewhere, so these are
particular meetings between doctors and parents circum-
scribed by time and place. Most of them occur or occurred
in a Scottish city over three and a half years in the
1970s; the rest took place over three weeks in an
American city of much the same size. Narrower still -
and three weeks seems narrow enough - these are primarily
meetings in the outpatient (or ambulatory) clinics of two
hospitals, though a few other kinds of encounter are
mentioned.

So now my title seems grandiose and even the sub-title
is inflated. (Would 'Three Weeks in Another Town' be
better?) Nevertheless there may be something in this
exaggeration, though justification will have to wait.

Sticking to the meetings - and I shall do this most of
the time - the point of my description is this: here are

over a thousand separate occasions on which parents met
doctors and met them in all kinds of different circumstances, and yet the manner of their meeting, the
ceremonial order of the occasion, was pretty much the
same no matter how other things might vary. One can go
further. The outward form of their relationship took just
the one shape, give or take a few minor alterations, in
all of the Scottish consultations and in most of the
American ones too.

So here we have something fairly powerful, a manner of
meeting, a mode of being doctor or parent, which was used
across a great range of contingencies and particularities;
this mode - the 'bureaucratic format' - is my main topic
and I shall try to describe its nature, its origins, the
methods by which it was sustained and the actual fit
between this outward show and the matters which it
clothed.

In doing all this I have several aims, some modest,
others less so. One is to comment on medical work with
children and their parents, another is to reflect more
generally on medical consultations, for although paediatrics is one small segment of the clinical world its
methods and dilemmas may well have their counterparts in
other areas of medicine. There may also be something for
sociologists. Medical consultations are merely one in a
myriad of those occasions and events which sociologists
study, and the frames or formats used therein may be of
little interest save to specialists in the field of
service relationships. Nevertheless, since the master
of ceremony, Erving Goffman himself, has paid little
attention to the study of any one order, the careful
delineation of a form may still have something to say
about formats in general and the structures which shape
our daily lives.

Acknowledgments

Unlike most modern products, sociology is normally
presented as the work of named individuals. Washing-
machines and cars may come to us with the names of their
makers attached, but we know that this is the name of an
organization, not of an individual. Our own machine is
merely one of thousands like it, in whose production
thousands are typically engaged. Further, the manner in
which this work-force is best co-ordinated is a topic of
constant public and theoretical concern. Sociology,
however, is often seen, even by its members, as a craft
where the quality of any individual piece of manufacture
is predominantly fixed by the skills of the craftsmen and
the intellectual tools with which he or she works. It is
to these features and not to the organization of the craft
that attention is typically directed. We focus on the
paradigm involved, which itself can hardly be said to
produce things, and on the specific arguments, which are
seen as representing the qualities of the individual
worker.

Moreover, even if we do inquire into the way this piece
of research came to be undertaken or that article written,
we experience great difficulty. For such information is
rarely given to us. We are presented merely with a
finished product whose most striking clue to its
production is the name of the author(s). The nearest
that we normally get to discovering the conditions under
which this product originated is a brief section, such as
this, called 'acknowledgments' and the address of an
institution in small print on the fly-leaf. Occasionally
a book may be found to be part of a series of such works,
all carried out at a particular institution. But such
information gives no clue as to how the work came into
being. The main focus still rests upon the author.

Such neglect is fostered by the craft nature of the

discipline. Not only do we 'see' authorship in others'
work but we experience it in our own. For, as members of
a cottage industry, we are typically in control of some
important aspects of our own production. We can often
determine the topic, the rate at which we work and the
occasions of our labour. Such personal control, particularly when contrasted with its absence in many other kinds
of work, can conceal some of the important constraints
that bind us. Although we can often exercise some choice
as to what we will produce, in practice almost all of us
have to choose from a very limited range of topics because
of the conditions of our employment as teachers or
researchers. Teachers find it hard to do field-work while
researchers, though they are certainly allowed, even
pushed into the field, often have little choice as to the
specific pasture or how long and in what fashion they may
graze.

At the same time, this individualization of the product
conceals not merely the constraints that bind the individual producer but the essential contribution made by
others. For intellectual goods are above all the products
of *conversation* and in this respect are co-authored by
one's colleagues and friends and those entrepreneurs who
create the intellectual and organizational climate in
which one works.

Clearly, one can do little in an acknowledgments
section to repair this gross omission. I have taken a
long time to produce this book and am indebted to a great
many people, many of whose contributions must remain
unacknowledged for there is little space in which to
mention them and little enough awareness on my own part
of the role which they have played. My first thanks must
go to those who persuaded me to move from teaching to
research and also to the SSRC (UK) which actually funded
the project on which this book is based, as part of a
programme grant to the Institute of Medical Sociology on
'Objectives and Needs in Systems of Social and Medical
Care'.

To all of my colleagues on the programme and at the
Institute I owe a great deal but particularly to Alan
Davis who not only gathered the data with me but has been
a source of invaluable ideas and conversation over many
years. Various drafts of the manuscript were typed
several times by Jeanette Thorn with speed, accuracy and
amazing good will. It was then read by Mildred Blaxter,
Alex Campbell, Robert Dingwall, Gordon Horobin, Raymond
Illsley, David May and Ross Mitchell, many of whose
comments I more or less grudgingly accepted. I am also
indebted to the medical staff of the various hospitals

and clinics who put up for so long with such an intrusion - as did the parents and their children. Since I have substituted letters for names and invented new ones where these appear in quotations, I cannot mention anyone directly but I would, in particular, like to thank Dr G, Dr I, Dr O and Dr N for all the help they gave me. Finally I owe an enormous amount to the advice, support and long-suffering nature of Gordon Horobin, Raymond Illsley and Angela Weight.

1 Introduction

One of the most striking features of modern life is the constant invention, application and modification of modes of formal organization. So endemic is this practice that we have a special name for those social entities that are most susceptible to this process. 'Organizations' are called after the techniques they most dramatically embody. Many of us work within formal organizations and all of us routinely encounter their representatives in our daily lives. However, although the social technology of the modern organization is as important as the industrial technology around which it is also based, it receives rather less publicity. Inventing the petrol engine has more status somehow than designing General Motors, if possibly smaller rewards. This is not to say that such matters are ignored, merely that the attention which is paid them is usually partial or specialist. Since this is so, the bureaucratization of medicine and its effects upon the doctor-patient relationship, or more generally staff-patient relationships, have received little attention. Much effort has been expended on examining some of the minutiae of these relationships, surprisingly little has gone on examining the context in which they occur. Without an understanding of that context and of the forces that produce it, many suggested reforms of medical practice will prove futile. This book does not itself set out to suggest such reforms. My aim is simply to provide information for their discussion.

Before considering my arguments in any detail it may prove useful to reflect on quite why the bureaucratic context of medical work has been ignored. First, much everyday discussion of organizations is often merely critical rather than analytic. In popular usage 'bureaucracy' and 'bureaucratic' have pejorative meanings rather than the purely technical ones that are standard

1

in sociology. 'Official' is a rather more neutral term
but it shades off into officious and officialdom, just as
formal organizational procedures become red tape. Even
'organization', which has a largely technical meaning, has
developed shades of menace, as in The Organization, and
facelessness, as in The Organization Man. In this lay
version, bureaucracies and bureaucrats are impersonal
entities against which individual human beings struggle
as best they can. It was somewhat in this fashion that
Stimson and Webb's (1975) sample of patients told each
other stories of their 'triumphs' over doctors. Similarly, the staff in this study had their moans about the
bureaucracies of which they were a part, but here 'the
bureaucrats' turned out to be someone other than themselves; the real villains were the administrators or
the booking and record staff.

The discussion in which such terms are used and
stories told is rarely systematic. A less critical and
more descriptive view of organizations may be found in
novels, television and films. Nevertheless, with a few
notable exceptions, for example 'Something Happened' by
Joseph Heller, or the films of Olmi, routine organizational life is largely ignored. The demands of television for
an endless supply of material have indeed generated series
that are based within organizations such as police departments, aircraft factories, prisons, motels and hospitals, and this genre has recently spread to popular novels
and films. However, with a few possible exceptions such
as the early programmes of 'Z-Cars', the organizations
are merely a backdrop for dramatic incident. Their
creators focus on bank robberies rather than petty theft,
on staff's romances, not on their alienation. Moreover,
just as the daily workings of these entities are ignored,
so too there is a similar absence of popular works about
the history of organizations. Most general readers of
history are more interested in the personal and biographi-
cal; in kings, queens and politicians. The only organizations which receive much written attention are military
ones and those such as ITT which have been implicated in
major political scandals.

There is, however, one popular form which does describe
the daily practice of organizations, the documentary, and
it is this which most closely approximates my intention
here. Filmed documentary has one powerful advantage.
The audience are shown the data with a vividness unmatched
by any other form of presentation. However, such a method
is analytically weak. As Galbraith has remarked, a
picture may sometimes be worth a thousand words, but the
reverse is often just as true. Ideally one should join

the two methods and in a more perfect world a book such as this would be accompanied by a film of some of the typical events that it describes.

For most people reflection upon organizations is a thing of the moment. For some it is their daily bread, and here at least we may find systematic analyses of the mysteries of organizational action. However, these too have their own particular biasses. The central weakness of much academic discussion of these matters is the polar opposite of that found in popular thought. Whereas the latter over-emphasizes individuals, scholarly debate commonly removes them altogether. The triumph of cog over machine, the drama of the operating table, the love between nurse and doctor; all these disappear. In their place stands the autonomous organization, independent of human will and action and vested with its own purposes and acts. In their concern to define and study organizations precisely, these writers have laid their entire stress on those formal procedures which separate organizations from other social entities and in doing so have reified bureaucracies, have turned them into things set totally apart from those who work within them (Bittner, 1965).

This reification is partly the product of the typical aims of such research. Managers and administrators and those whom they sponsor, whether directly or indirectly, to engage in research are all largely preoccupied with the efficiency of organizational functioning. Monitoring and evaluation are the key tasks and organizational modification the end. However, these concerns would seem to have a differential effect upon the students of bureaucracy. Academic outsiders tend to reify the organizations which they study, but those involved in daily struggle within them are prone to a somewhat different fault. In this second version, and it is this which dominates the discussion of medical work with patients, the central concept in understanding bureaucracies is 'communication' (Ley and Spelman, 1967; Fletcher, 1973, Bennett, 1976; Byrne and Long, 1976). Whereas in the academic model the organization is reduced to a series of formal procedures, here these aspects disappear and emphasis is placed upon relationships between individuals. In this it has something in common with the lay tradition mentioned earlier. However, unlike this, its principal stress is on consensus not conflict, on reaching understanding not on achieving victory. The lay tradition emphasizes intensely personal feelings and interests, with the organization a mere locale for their expression, but these exist in the communications model only in so far as they are held to be organizationally relevant. Po-

litically, the model is espoused by the liberal and
counter-posed to what are seen as old-fashioned formality
and unquestionable hierarchy; and in many ways it presents a critical, reforming approach to professional work.
At the same time, it upholds and undoubtedly stems from
that central ethic of the profession which emphasizes
service to the individual client.

This emphasis on individuals leads to a stress on
personalities, perceptions and individual style. Staff
are instructed to inspect their own actions, to be nicer
and more understanding towards their patients. Harsh,
intolerant action is condemned, and so is the unthinking
and routine. Staff are also exhorted to learn more about
the different personal and cultural backgrounds of their
clients, and there may also be pressure for professional
recruitment to reflect this diversity. At the same time
such analysts are sensitive to the problems, opinions,
satisfactions and dissatisfactions of their patients.
Interview studies of patients are a favourite vehicle for
combining both these approaches. On the one hand they may
reveal something of their background and expectations; on
the other hand they give them a chance to express their
opinions on the service they have received. Finally,
great awareness is displayed of the many possible misunderstandings that may occur between staff and patients.
The research that is done here pays special attention to
how staff and patients actually talk to each other. Its
emphasis is on listening more carefully to what people
say, using a language they will understand, and so on.

The principal reform that is urged by such writers is
better education. They seek the modification of the
medical school curriculum and may even themselves provide
means for re-education. Byrne and Long (1976) not only
organize conferences at which general practitioners may
learn new communications skills, but also provide a home
tutor in these. There is much that is beneficial in such
an approach and yet, as Freidson notes, it suffers from
the faults of all individualist thought:

> In considering how the members of the profession work
> its leaders typically see solutions to the problem of
> poor or unethical work in recruiting better-motivated
> and more capable entrants to school, in improving their
> professional education and in generally 'raising
> standards'. All these devices are predicated on the
> aim of changing the quality of *individuals,* the as-
> sumption being first that social pathologies connected
> with medical care, like illnesses connected with
> mankind, are 'caused' by the characteristics of the

individual providing the care rather than by the
environment in which those individuals provide care,
and second that they are best treated by treating the
individual rather than the environment (Freidson,
1970b, p.6).

In other words, the communications approach, by
emphasizing the individual, renders the organization
itself transparent; its actual workings, organizational
procedures and resources, the social settings and roles
of the participants, all of these are simply assumed. At
the same time, despite this atomization of individual
members, organizational purposes are still present but in
covert and thus uninspected form. Individuals are viewed
not in their own terms, not in the light of their actual
interests, commitments, resources and constraints, but
solely as regards the official goals of the organization.
Thus 'communication' is used in a very special sense. It
does not refer to all the myriad ways in which doctor and
patient both present their behaviour and read that of the
other as each attempt to make sense of and to control the
situation, but simply means seeing that illness is efficiently diagnosed and patients properly informed about
their illnesses.
    Similarly, although there is a search for disharmony
and an attempt to put it right, such matters are regarded
as purely surface features, for there is a basic assumption that the interests of staff and patients are one
and the same. Patients want to be cured, staff wish to
cure them. Most conflict or dissatisfaction is viewed as
a product of misunderstanding or mistaken technique and
not of anything more fundamental.
    My own position emphasizes the structural context in
which individual action occurs. If one wishes to explain
behaviour or seeks to modify it, it is as important to
look to the system as it is to the individuals who work
within it. At the same time I take a rather more pessi-
mistic view of organizations than is held by those who
write within the communications tradition. As I shall
argue, there are fundamental and irreconcilable conflicts
inherent within medical consultations, and these occur,
not just between staff and parents, but even within the
various things that any one individual may want or have
to do. We seek to solve these dilemmas as best we can
and may at various times try out a variety of solutions,
but each entails its own problems and none is more than
provisional - though some may prove more satisfactory
than others.

MEDICAL ROLE-RELATIONSHIPS

My own aim is to render the transparent apparent, to set
the business of diagnosis, treatment and their discussion
within an organizational framework. There are various
ways in which this might be done and mine is only one of
these and a highly restricted one at that. My concern is
with the consultation itself and more specifically with
its overt social form. The question I have asked of each
consultation is: what kind of social occasion is this?
When we ask this question normally, we refer to something
rather special and out of the ordinary. A 'social
occasion' is seen as more formal, more public and more
artificial than everyday events. To be at one is to be
on display and thus hopefully on one's best behaviour.
One needs to know in advance just what the rules are:
what one should wear; what may and may not be said; and
to whom one may talk and when. And yet, seen from another
perspective, all social intercourse shares these qualities, if to a less self-conscious degree. Whenever we
talk to someone we are in one sense on display. Judgments
about our character and competence are routinely made by
others as we in turn judge them. The smallest detail of
speech, tone, posture or dress can serve as evidence in
this, and may accordingly be adjusted to suit the
occasion. Thus, all social life has an artificial, rule-
governed and ceremonial aspect (and may thus be seen as
artfully constructed), though many of our calculations
are so routine that they pass unnoticed even by ourselves.
It is this ceremony that I am principally concerned with
and, in a phrase, my topic is the 'ritual' aspect of
medical consultations. (1)
    As we shall see, there are special sets of rules that
make medical consultations distinct social occasions,
rules that are clearly informed by the location of the
action within a bureaucratic setting. In claiming that
this occasion has a distinct form, I do not deny that
there are important differences between one consultation
and another. Some recent researchers who have observed
medical consultations have emphasized the differences
between doctors. Byrne and Long (1976) have noted
distinct personal styles with respect to the role that
doctors let patients play in the consultation. At a more
microscopic level, Bloor (1976a, 1976b) has demonstrated
that in one condition at least, tonsillitis, different
consultants use very different criteria and search procedures in their decision-making. Consultations will also
differ according to the patient, the medical condition,
and the particular setting in which the patient is seen.

The research reported here was done in collaboration with
Alan Davis, whose own work (1978) has focussed on the
distinct variation produced by the different tasks which
different clinics set for the doctor. Yet, despite all
this variation it still makes sense to talk of a general
form, or rather forms, which medical consultations hold
in common, something over and above these other differences, and which distinguishes them from, say, taking
one's car to a garage or buying groceries at a supermarket. (2)

These forms, as I argued earlier, have received relatively little empirical attention. The two studies worthy
of note are those of Parsons (1951) and Stimson and Webb
(1975). Parsons's study was in fact carried out in the
1930s but it was not written up until many years later.
It utilized the classic sociological concept for ex-
pressing the differences between social occasions, the
theatrical metaphor of role. In this, each person is
seen as having a repertoire of different parts, some of
which are common to all, others of which are more specialist. Parsons described two roles in medical consultations, the role of the patient - the 'sick role' - and
the corresponding role of the doctor; the two together
equalling the 'doctor-patient role relationship'. His
analysis has been extremely influential but since it is
highly complex, being in fact part of a much wider attempt
to explain all social life, it will not be considered in
detail here. (3)

Suffice it to say that there are several parallels
between the analysis presented in this book and that of
Parsons. Both models emphasize the doctor's technical
authority over the patient, and the impersonality and
neutrality of medical interaction. At the same time
Parsons's analysis has serious flaws. Although it was
derived from both observation and interview, the research
itself is not specified and no data are presented to
warrant the assertions made, a drawback which is all the
more considerable given the very high level of generality
at which Parsons writes. He also assumes that there is
only the one role-relationship between doctor and patient,
that the social form is always the same. This, as will be
shown later, is a gross mistake and one which arises in
part from the ahistorical nature of the analysis. Parsons
fails to link his description of the rules of doctor-
patient interaction to the specific structural, ideological and organizational context. There is little sense
in his work that doctors are doing a job under specific
sets of conditions which severely constrain the work they
perform.

The general model of interaction which Parsons uses, that of role analysis, is severely defective. In one sense role theorists have taken the theatrical analogy too far. They write as if there were detailed, pre-ordained scripts which players learnt off by heart and then repeated, word for word, on relevant occasions. They omit the sense in which social occasions are continuously constructed by their participants. There are indeed rules to be followed but there are often many different ways in which this may be done, and one rule may conflict with another. Moreover, rules are used as well as followed, but role theoristsomit the conflictual and strategic aspects of interaction. For Parsons, moral neutrality, medical control and impersonality are simply written into the script. He fails to see that achieving them and using them for whatever purposes one has presents serious and complex problems to the participants.

Although many of Stimson and Webb's conclusions about the form of the occasion are in some respects similar to those reached by Parsons, they are more adequately demonstrated and are set in a far more convincing general model of interaction, that provided by Goffman. (4) However, just as Parsons's main interest was the formulation of a general theory of society and not the study of consultations, so for Stimson and Webb the social form of medical relationships is a backdrop to their principal theme. Their main story concerns the patients, not the social form, and they are interested in patients' expectations of a medical consultation, their strategies during it, and their consequent behaviour and opinions. Therefore they do not set out to provide a detailed model of the doctor-patient role-relationship, while their relatively brief reflections upon it are based on only a limited amount of data: they observed fifty consultations in two group practices run by general practitioners.

There is therefore scope for a detailed study of the social forms of medical consultations. Such forms I shall call 'role formats', although I will not stick unswervingly to this terminology and to avoid the endless repetition of the term I shall substitute phrases such as 'mode', 'model' or 'framework' on occasion. In the consultations reported on here, there were four types of role format in use, which I have named the 'bureaucratic', 'charity', 'clinical' and 'private' modes respectively. (5)

With these formats I am concerned, almost exclusively, with doctor-parent interaction. By and large the matters to be considered here do not directly involve children. At first, it may seem odd for a study of medical work with children to exclude any systematic consideration of

the children themselves or of adults' relationship with
them. If this study were of a ward or concentrated
entirely on therapists' work with children, then such
puzzlement would indeed be justified. In such studies
children played a central part in the interaction; and,
as Alan Davis and I (1976a) have shown, medical work took
on a special shape to accommodate this. (6) But in
outpatient clinics things were different. In all but two
cases, the child had an adult representative, someone who
could act on his or her behalf, someone who in fact took
over most of the patient role within the consultation.
It was the parents or guardians who owned, managed and
worried about the children's future; and it was to them,
as the children's representatives, that talk was normally
addressed. For almost all children, even the older ones,
were routinely and smoothly excluded from the bulk of the
action within most consultations; the adults present,
both staff and parents, used a wide range of devices to
this end.

Thus, the reason for my exclusion of children from this
book is that they themselves were largely excluded from
the consultations. Quite how this exclusion was managed
will be considered in chapter 8. For the moment I shall
merely note its occurrence.

My topic, then, is the formats used between doctors
and parents; and of the various modes that were in use
I have selected just one, the bureaucratic format, as the
principal object for analysis because it was by far the
most commonly observed form. Despite the striking differences between the principles that underlay the Scottish
and American medical services, this one mode was found in
almost all settings. It was in universal, though not
always sole use in the Scottish hospital, and was the most
frequent mode in the American hospital. Even in clinics
where other formats were used, it was still the typical
mode.

Note that in calling it the bureaucratic format I am
not suggesting that it has all the characteristics which
are popularly ascribed to bureaucracies. The particular
form that I describe here is subtle and complex, and one
that might not spring immediately to mind if one was asked
to speculate on the shape that medical bureaucracy might
take in consultations. For this reason, the greater part
of the book is devoted to an explication of its various
rules and their use in differing circumstances. Only at
the end do I suggest reasons for their existence and
discuss how far my analysis may be generalized to other
medical work.

Note also that although the bureaucratic mode will

receive most of my attention, I shall at times pay close
regard to certain aspects of the other formats. My aim
is not to engage in any systematic study of these other
modes, for I have little enough data on some of them;
rather it is to bring out the special nature of the
bureaucratic format by highlighting particularly striking
differences from other modes. My analyses of the latter
are meant to serve as signposts to the bureaucratic
format, not as detailed maps to their own interior.

THE CONCEPT OF ROLE FORMAT

Before proceeding to outline the research on which this
analysis is based, it may be useful to outline my underlying theoretical stance and to spell out in a little more
detail just what is meant by role format, though non-
sociologists may prefer to skip this section.
    Given my concern with the ceremonial aspects of medical
interaction, I am heavily dependent on the work of the
leading analyst of everyday ritual, Erving Goffman (1961,
1963,1970,1971a,1971b,1972,1975a,1975b). However, the
central concept in this monograph, that of role format,
is not to be found in Goffman's own writings, but is one
of my own invention. Goffman has produced so many new
concepts in his time that I thought I might try my own
hand at this game and besides, despite his great prolifer-
ation of conceptual aids, none of the relevant terms which
he offers quite fits my own purposes, though what I myself
have to suggest is merely an offshoot or close relative of
Goffman's own classifications. The fundamentals of
Goffman's analysis are described by Gonos in the following
fashion:

> Everyday life is seen to be made up of more or less
> well-delineated 'worlds', realms of special meaning
> within which a particular language of reality is
> binding. The world is a mode of experience fleshed
> out by adherence to the rules of a frame or occasion
> ... a frame is described by the stable rules of its
> operation, whatever the circumstances of any particular
> enactment. In other words, frames are not to be
> thought of as empirical in the way that situations are
> (Gonos, 1977, p.857).

> What guides conduct in this structuralist world is not
> a set of shady core values or the influence of others
> who are co-present, but the individual's place within
> the formal social organization of a concrete social

activity, or to put it differently, one's place with
respect to the social relations of production of a
ritual world (Gonos, 1977, p.862).

Grasping Goffman's own classification of these frames
is a rather difficult task, since he has written volumi-
nously in and around the area but has never supplied any
ordered guide to his own work. New terms and new ideas
are continually appearing and the relation of any one to
any other is a matter for some speculation. Moreover, he
himself has not been interested in depicting the particularities of any individual social forms, save those of
games and of the theatre, both of which are rather special
kinds of frame set apart from the more serious business of
daily life.

Three broad distinctions between types of frame can,
however, be discerned in Goffman's work. The first of
these is a division of frames into two fundamental
classes, those which are seen as applying to 'natural'
events and those which are used for 'social' phenomena
(Goffman, 1975a). Among social frames there is in turn
a crucial distinction between 'focussed' and 'unfocussed'
gatherings, that is between those which apply when people
are merely in one another's presence and those which
regulate occasions when there is a single focus of cognitive and visual attention. These latter occasions are
termed 'encounters' or 'situated activity systems'
(Goffman, 1961). Finally Goffman distinguishes between
different types of encounter, between those which are
merely one-off affairs and those which develop an institutionalized form:

When the runs of a situated system are repeated with
any frequency, fairly well-developed *situated roles*
seem to emerge: action comes to be divided into
manageable bundles, each a set of acts that can be
compatibly performed by a single participant. In
addition to this role formation, there is a tendency
for role differentiation to occur, so that the package
of activity that the members of one class perform is
different from, though dependent upon, the set performed by members of another category. These kinds of
roles, it may be added, differ from roles in general,
not only because they are realized and encompassed in
a face-to-face situation but also because the pattern
of which they are a part can be confidently identified
as a concrete, self-compensating system (Goffman, 1961,
p.96).

With this final distinction we have at last a unit of
analysis which is appropriate to the interaction considered in this study. Medical consultations are clearly
institutionalized activity systems, encounters that are
repeated over and over again, though not always by the
same participants or in the same settings. Moreover there
is, as I shall show, a complex division of labour which
sustains a joint version of reality across such a wide
diversity of individual circumstances that the frame can,
with some truth, be seen as self-compensating.

Goffman's own attempt to encompass the ceremonial order
of such frames, the notion of 'situated role', is clearly
inadequate, and represents a partial throwback to the
traditional versions of role theory. He writes as if
there was only one situated role for each participant in
an activity system, thus repeating the classic mistake of
assuming that there was only one role for each and every
status. This was certainly not true of the medical
consultations discussed here where a variety of frames
were in use; for the precise way in which an activity is
framed is historically situated and changes according to
different circumstance. The definitions of reality
embodied in a particular frame are both shaped by and
enforce a particular balance of power. Indeed, political
dispute is precisely centred around the proper content of
frames: what is or is not the correct way of doing this
or that activity. To presume that for every activity
there is one and only one frame is to re-enter that
timeless, unchanging and apolitical world of functionalism
from which sociology has spent so much effort trying to
escape. Roles are not situated in quite this sense. (7)

Aside from these political considerations, there is
also a point which concerns the priority of individuals
or frames in frame analysis. By itself, a concept such
as situated role gives undue prominence to one individual's share in any particular ceremonial order and detracts
from the sense in which an institutionalized order forms a
coherent whole. What is needed then is a concept which
refers to the entire ceremonial order and it is this which
I have termed 'role format'. Situated roles still have a
place in this analysis but they are merely components of a
larger unity.

It should not be thought that the notion of a role
format means a narrow determinism, with each and every
action constrained to fit a particular social order. Far
from it. Although such a concept helps to capture the
heavily structured nature of social life it is also meant
to avoid the over-determinism typical of traditional role
analysis. A role format supplies merely a guideline for

the overt form of events, not a detailed prescription;
indeed, more than one role format may be used in an
encounter. Further, since role formats are concerned
primarily with the outer show, with overt and not covert
behaviour, all manner of things may be done so long as
they are decently clothed. Thus, although such forms are
based on and originate in a particular balance of interests and resources, they can in fact accommodate quite
wide variation within these. They constitute a resource
to which all kinds of problem may be brought for solution,
so long, that is, as the participants agree. In essence,
role formats are not structures which totally determine
action but are instead routinized, culturally available
solutions which members 'use' to solve whatever problems
they have at hand. (8)

All this is not to say that we are free to do whatever
we like. In any particular encounter, actions are constrained by the following circumstances: by the interests
and resources of the participants; by the range of role
formats available to them; by the identities and actions
that these permit; by the extent to which other participants share a common interest in the use of particular
role formats; by one's relative ability to enforce an
agreed practical meaning of the constituent rules of a
format; and finally, by the extent to which participants
are accountable to outsiders for their actions, are
visible by the same and are in some way dependent upon
them. As these features vary so the participants in some
encounters may be relatively free to do what they like,
while in others they may be severely constrained. The
encounters to be considered here fall into the latter
category, but even here there was still considerable
flexibility compared with the rigid prescription of
action as formulated in traditional role studies.

A DESCRIPTION OF THE RESEARCH

The data on which my analysis is based were gathered over
a three-and-a-half-year period in some of the paediatric
services of two cities of roughly comparable size, one
Scottish and the other American. The Scottish city formed
the principal location. Within these two cities, the
paediatric and therapy services of the two children's
hospitals were the main objects of attention, but study
was also given to the children's clinics run by the city
and state authorities. During the study 1,120 consultations were observed between staff, patients and parents,
all but 100 of these within the Scottish settings. Apart

from this, observation was also carried out at a number of consultations where only staff and child patients were present. Almost all of these occurred in the ward-round at an intensive care unit for newborn babies in the maternity hospital in the Scottish city.

The principal method of data-collection was that of verbatim note-taking. Two researchers gathered the data, Alan Davis and myself. Typically we stood or sat to one side of the consultation, often with medical students, and made a written record of what was said and done. (In only one setting did this not apply: in the American city children's clinic accounts of the cases were written up from memory immediately afterwards.) All these written notes were then taped and transcribed. Apart from this observational data, interviews were carried out with those staff who had been studied most intensively. Doctors often engaged in informal discussion about the work of clinics in the intervals between consultations, sometimes with the researchers, and sometimes with other staff or students. This too was noted, taped and transcribed.

The extent to which particular conditions, settings, patients, parents and staff were studied varied considerably. Nevertheless, the data were sufficiently extensive to allow a wide range of internal comparisons to be made in testing the universality of the rules under investigation. Further details of the settings and of the data are given in chapter 2. At this point the following features of the data seem worthy of particular attention.

First, one setting, the Scottish neurological clinic, was studied continuously over a three-year period. This provided an opportunity to study the relationship between doctors, patients and parents as it developed over time, in contrast to the purely cross-sectional data available from the other settings. At the extreme, one child was observed 12 times in the neurological clinic, and three others were seen on nine separate occasions. Three years is by no means the limit of a patient career in an outpatient department, for many will require medical attention all their lives. Nevertheless, this period of observation provided a useful insight into the more long-term relationships and the way they developed.

A second relevant feature of consultations was the great variation in their length. Some lasted no more than a minute, a few took over an hour. A great range of medical conditions was also seen. (This is discussed more fully in chapter 2.) A fourth source of variation lay in the number of staff observed. In all, the work of 40 doctors and 12 therapists was studied, although the number of staff considered in any detail was rather less.

In essence, this book is about the work of 9 Scottish
doctors, 5 Scottish therapists and 4 American doctors,
but even though far fewer data were gathered on other
staff, these have none the less provided a useful check
on the main body. Fifth, just as there was considerable
variation in the types of patient and parent observed in
most settings, so too an attempt was made to study a
variety of doctors in any one setting or type of setting.
Thus, at one extreme five Scottish local authority doctors
were studied.

Some data were also gathered on the same patient in
different settings. This formed a sixth type of comparison, though very few such cases were seen. In all, 27
children were observed in more than one Scottish setting,
21 of these in just two locales and the remaining six in
three others. The great majority of these cases were
patients at the neurological clinic who were also being
treated in one of the therapy departments, or else
children who were receiving simultaneous treatment at
both occupational therapy and physiotherapy. Turning to
the number of settings involved in the study, observations
were made in 24 types of locale, though only a few of
these were studied in detail. Once again the American
data inflate this number considerably. In the principal
area of study, the Scottish city, only 9 types of locale
were studied.

The American data, though small by comparison and
stretched across a wide range of staff and settings,
nevertheless provided a valuable series of comparisons,
for there are major differences between the Scottish and
American medical systems and these provided two contrasting sets of possible variables.

Such a list demonstrates the considerable width and
depth of the data. However, the following negative
features should in justice also be noted. First,
interview data were gathered only from the doctors, not
from the parents or children, though a separate interview
study with the parents of 40 children from the neurological clinic was carried out by Heather Gibson. (This had
as its main focus a somewhat more specialized topic, the
medical experience of handicapped children.) Second, the
outpatient work of only two children's hospitals was
examined, and one of these in only the briefest of detail.
Third, the data are almost exclusively concerned with
paediatricians and therapists. Yet there are many other
medical specialities to be found in children's hospitals,
specialities which may well have different traditions or
different technical constraints. Fourth, the range of
specialisms within paediatrics itself was by no means

covered. Fifth, as a result of these last two omissions
certain extremes to be found in medical work are not
present. The severe problems presented by handicap were
certainly studied in detail; but very high technology
medicine as found, say, in specialist paediatric cardiology units is not represented (see Hilliard *et al.*,
1977). Nor, on the other hand, is the most heavily
routinized work considered, such as routine decision-
making concerning adeno-tonsillectomy (see Bloor, 1976a,
1976b).

FOUR PRE-EMPTIVE MANOEUVRES

Finally, some doubts may arise concerning the adequacy of
my procedures for gathering and analysing the data on
which this study is based. Does observation alter
people's behaviour so radically that such accounts are
worthless? Can such data be quantified and, if not, what
value are they? Is it possible to grasp the meaning of
action in any adequate fashion given what we all know
about ambiguity, indexicality, self-deception and error?
Are there any coherent procedures for the generation and
testing of hypotheses in qualitative data? Such worries
may be of no concern. In which case, read on. For the
more cynical or technically-minded some discussion of my
answer to these questions may be found in an appendix.
    But not everything can be so readily assigned to
oblivion, for some prior comments must be made concerning
the fairness of my account. The first concerns my terminology. Words such as 'bourgeois' or 'bureaucratic' are
intended in a technical, sociological sense and should not
be read as condemning the phenomena which they describe.
Likewise, my choice of names for the other formats is not
meant to convey any particular approval or disapproval of
their nature. The bureaucratic format is so called simply
because it displays many of the classical features
ascribed by sociologists to bureaucracies, while its use
was so nearly universal within the medical bureaucracies
that were studied that this name seemed more appropriate
than any other.
    Second, some of the methods used to demonstrate the
existence, nature and scope of the rules of the bureaucratic format lead to a concentration on the extreme and
the atypical. Thus, it should not be assumed that the
quotations I provide are totally representative of the
general run of behaviour in clinics; and in this sense
the book is misleading. But this emphasis on the abnormal
is not a mere pandering to exotica. For my purpose, which

is the demonstration of the existence of certain rules, it is the unusual which very often has the greatest technical relevance. As I have argued in the appendix, it may be the only means by which the nature of the rules may be brought home fully to the reader.

Some unease may arise through my constant contrasting of overt and covert action. The comparison of what we say in private with what we say in public is commonly used to make a moral point, to reveal the hypocrisy of the speaker and the occasion; but such debunking is far from my intention. It is central to my argument that people necessarily say one thing here and another thing there, that types of discourse are appropriate to the occasion. In consequence they should not be judged by standards imported from different contexts. I am not arguing that there should be one standard for all occasions, or that staff or parents were hypocrites and liars. One may quarrel with the exclusion of particular matters from a particular ceremonial order, but to assert that any exclusion is in principle bad is to ignore the reality of the way all social interaction is actually conducted. Social life depends upon a tacit agreement to concentrate on some things and ignore others. (9)   My emphasis on the ceremonial order of consultations serves merely to display the complex social rules which any competent participant is normally obliged to observe. Similarly, in comparing overt and covert action, I aim simply to reveal what is and is not said and to show the difficulties that are caused by the inclusion or exclusion of particular topics.

This mere exposition may at times seem to 'expose' those whom I have studied, and this is particularly true of the medical staff; for while I have extensive data on the public actions of both doctors and parents my data on their more private thoughts or deeds are asymmetrical. I have considerable evidence of the more covert feelings and actions of staff, but far less which concerns those of parents. Although more data on the latter would obviously have been desirable, their absence presents no major technical difficulties. My principal topic is the overt order, while since it is staff who principally control the interaction, their covert actions are of greater analytical significance than those of parents. Although this asymmetry does not seriously threaten the credibility of the argument, it may at times serve to show staff in rather a poor light. Whereas I can quote doctors who said one thing to parents but said the opposite as soon as they had left the clinic, I cannot do the same for parents, although no doubt they regularly behaved in a similar fashion. To those who are offended by any of this I apologize.

2 Medical systems and settings

Summary descriptions of institutions and rapid surveys of the sources of one's data normally engender a creeping paralysis in the unfortunate reader. Here, alas, there seems no way round it. Without some mention of my data I have no warrant for my analysis; without a sketch of the various clinics and the medical systems of which they were a part the reader will make little sense of what I have to say.

The description of the settings has in fact a treble purpose. It serves to familiarize the reader with the background to my story, so that the individual scenes described later become somewhat easier to visualize. But it is also an essential part of the telling of that story, for one of my main themes, the use of the bureaucratic format across a wide variety of circumstances, can be appreciated only if one has some knowledge of those circumstances. At the same time, some background knowledge of organizational structure and setting is essential when considering the origins of both the bureaucratic format and of the other formats mentioned here.

A GENERAL COMPARISON BETWEEN THE SCOTTISH AND AMERICAN SYSTEMS

I shall begin the task of scene-setting with the broadest possible brush and contrast the Scottish and American health systems, or at least those aspects of them which are most relevant to my purposes. (1) Although I have relatively little data on the services for children in the American city, the very striking differences in the system of which it was a part may bring some of the essential features of the NHS into much sharper focus. I shall describe first the Scottish services.

Broadly speaking, the aim of the Scottish health system
was to provide services for the entire population, and it
was in fact used by almost all of that population.   Four
main principles are crucial to an understanding of its
workings.   First, it was a self-consciously organized
system which was planned, in certain vital respects, as
an ordered whole in which each part had its special place.
Thus the Scottish city had just one children's hospital,
which in principle handled all the serious medical conditions affecting any child in the city (apart that is
from infectious diseases, which were seen at another
hospital which had isolation facilities).   Certain
services did overlap in some respects, such as the well-
baby clinics and the general practitioners.   There were
also some demarcation disputes: for example, as between
occupational therapy and physiotherapy, and between
paediatrics and orthopaedics.   Nevertheless, there were
key structuring principles which maintained an order
between all the various parts:
a Patients 'belonged' to the general practitioner with
whom they were registered.   Local authority doctors had
no authority to prescribe or treat and could refer
patients to hospital only via general practitioners.
Each time they saw a patient, hospital doctors were
obliged to send a letter to the general practitioner
describing what they had done.
b Doctors were crucially divided between generalists,
who worked in general practice, and specialists who worked
in hospitals.   Since the former had only a general
training and had limited technical resources they were
obliged to refer their more serious or difficult cases to
hospitals.
c Patient access to the system was heavily controlled.
Patients could have one and only one general practitioner
(though in a group practice they might well be treated by
more than one of the partners).   Only general practitioners could refer patients to hospital.   Self-referral was
not allowed, except to 'Casualty'.   Similarly within the
hospital, referral, both as between departments and as
between different hospitals, was controlled by staff.
Patients did, however, have the right to ask for a second
opinion.
d There was an elaborate body of governing committees
at both local and national level which mediated disputes
between sections and which was responsible for the formulation of policy and the provision of finance.
The second principle for understanding the Scottish
system is that the means of financing the service were
provided almost entirely by the state, and that finance

was conceived of at an organizational level rather than in
terms of individual transactions between professional and
patient. Although all employed citizens paid a 'contribution' to the health services as a separate tax upon
their income, and although part of the local property tax,
'rates', went to finance the local authority health department, nevertheless the greater part of health expendi-
ture came directly out of central government funds. Just
as crucially, the accounting systems normally took no
notice of individual medical transactions. That is, it
was not just that medicine was 'free' but that there was
no 'fee-for-service' paid either by the state or by
insurance companies. (This avoided the enormous paper-
work commonly associated with this method.) Doctors'
income was fixed not by their patients but by national
criteria negotiated through their professional association.

Third, the services were available to all those
domiciled in the country, and were routinely used by
all but a tiny fraction of the population. The clinics
that were observed treated the children of academics and
American oil-workers, local businessmen and local aristocracy, as well as those of farm-labourers and tinkers,
the unskilled and the unemployed.

Finally, although the majority of services were simply
there and available to anyone who turned up, a few were
enforced upon the population as far as was possible. The
hospital obstetricians and paediatricians had worked
closely with the city health department in trying to
monitor and control every pregnancy and every young child
in the city. All confinements were hospital confinements.
All newborn babies could therefore be screened at birth
and all were followed up at clinics - or at least the
attempt was made. Where they did not appear health
visitors pursued them in their homes, and central registers were kept of children who needed special attention.
Great pride was taken in the efficiency and effectiveness
of these operations, and great upset was caused if a child
with a clear impairment slipped through the net. (2)

By contrast the American system was based, not on an
ordered division of labour but on its opposite, a free
market philosophy. Different medical units were in open
competition with each other. Although there was only one
children's hospital in the city, there were several other
hospitals which had children's wards and there was considerable competition between these to attract the more
lucrative patients. In those specialisms where it was
particularly strong, the children's hospital also competed
with hospitals in other areas of the state and indeed

across the whole region of the United States in which it
was situated.

At the same time, there was no such clear division
between generalists and specialists, between individual
practitioners and hospitals as was found in the Scottish
system. Thus, there was no distinction between primary
and secondary levels of care, and patients could refer
themselves to hospital if they so chose. In consequence,
although the American children's hospital was in some ways
far more specialized than its Scottish counterpart
(concentrating heavily on orthopaedics) it also saw
patients who would have been treated entirely by their
general practitioner if they had been in Scotland. At
the same time, many individual practitioners were specialists themselves and either had important technical facilities of their own, or else, or in addition, used those of
the local hospital. Thus, there was a tradition of hospitals being staffed by individual practitioners - called
'attendings'. Hospitals in this classic version were
little more than locales with technical facilities to
which individual practitioners brought their patients when
necessary. Where other types of specialist were required
this was an individual deal between the private patient,
the doctor and the other specialist.

The range of choice available to patients was therefore
extremely wide compared to that in Scotland, at least in
theory. In practice, of course, only the rich could
exercise this freedom with ease. As Roth (1977) has
argued, even the middle classes in America are beginning
to be restricted to set health service organizations
through the increasing use of pre-paid schemes such as
Kaiser-Permanente. For the poor there was little choice,
and for them many of the services rendered by general
practitioners in Scotland were filled, after a fashion,
by the casualty departments of the large city hospitals
(Roth, 1975). Since the main organizing principle was
financial, there were many sick children in whom the
various private organizations had little interest, since
their parents had no money. Only the rich were worth
competing for. In consequence a variety of agencies
attempted to fill some of the gaps. One of the other
hospitals in the city had a large research grant to study
neonates, and ran a free baby clinic to attract subjects.
A local ethnic organization also ran a children's clinic,
as did the city itself.

These other services did more than fill gaps. They
also added a further element of competition. The complex
ways in which this worked is best seen by examining one
service, the Crippled Children's Service, which was

jointly funded by federal and state government for the benefit of the poor. Normally, this money was given direct to the state government to run its own service. However, in this particular instance the greater part of the funds went to the children's hospital studied here, even though it was a private institution. In return it agreed to offer its services to the local poor. The government service therefore provided clinics only in the more distant parts of the state. In this respect it had lost out to the powerful private hospital and faced yet further threats elsewhere. For example, one of its clinics was under pressure from another hospital in which it was temporarily located. If this hospital saw the patients directly and cut out the state service, then it would receive the federal and state money instead. In other words, the various medical units such as practitioners or hospitals competed, not simply for the fees of individual patients, but for income from any source whatsoever, whether city, state or federal schemes. Thus the financing of what were 'private' institutions often contained a very large proportion of public money.

This welter of competing institutions was not without various forms of regulation. At one level there were federal and state laws. (The poverty of the state medical department meant that its principal function was a licensing one — approving this or that hospital or clinic — though in fact it had never yet withdrawn a licence.) At another level the insurance companies, the principal means through which the better-off paid for their medicine, were taking an increasing interest in the efficiency or at least the cost of medical services. The children's hospital had begun to modify various of its practices in line with pressure from these companies. There was also some internal ordering of the market in progress. At the suggestion of the local medical school a cartel had recently been formed by the various hospitals in order to remove the more extravagant results of competition such as the duplication of cardiac surgery units. Finally, the last few years had seen a trend towards the creation of a full-time body of hospital staff, although the extent to which this had occurred varied. There was only one 'attending' left on the paediatric side of the children's hospital, but rather more on the orthopaedic side.

Despite these various attempts at rationalization, the system was still fundamentally competitive. This produced several important contrasts with the Scottish system, as regards both the public style of individual organizations and the quality of care at both individual and community levels.

Since each American organization was in the market-
place, each tried to establish a distinct public image
and each displayed the certificates which warranted it a
proper institution in a prominent public place. In one
way or another each organization had a product to sell,
even if the rewards were sometimes political and not
economic. The city children's clinic, for instance, was
decorated with large photographs showing members of
different ethnic groups going about their daily rounds,
shopping, eating and talking. The style of these images
was morally uplifting. Apparently the community was one
and the city fathers cared. The main city hospital, again
a public institution, had a large board in its entrance
hall on which were numbered the babies born that day and
the inpatients currently in residence. (How many had just
died was not announced.) The children's hospital, a
private institution, was also decorated with photographs,
wistful or joyous children in this case. It too stressed
its own special qualities. It had its own flag; visitors
were shown round on guided tours; and brochures told of
its special qualities:

City Children's Hospital is widely recognized throughout the state and the nation as an outstanding medical
facility.... Unlike most other children's hospitals,
patients are received from birth and continue through
age 21 so that the effects of growth and maturation,
both in the physical and psychosocial sense, takes
place with continuity in the total care and management
of the child.

Its Public Relations Department stressed the loving care
of the staff, and the pioneering advances they had made.
The theme of 'service' was a central one, and the hospital's official goals were spelled out for its customers
and backers in the following terms: 'care and treatment
for children without restriction to race, colour, creed,
sex, national origin or financial status.'
By contrast, the various institutions in the Scottish
city had a faceless character. They did not issue pro-
spectuses or state their goals for all to see. That each
organization cared for all, regardless of race, colour,
creed or income bracket might have been assumed, but it
was not stated. The children's hospital had a sign
outside which gave its name but that was all. 'It was
apparently just a children's hospital, much like one might
find anywhere else in the country. There was no literature which proclaimed its strengths or special nature, and
no photographs or certificates hung on the walls. Simi-

larly, although the Scottish city authorities took great
pride in their health services, such pride was not made
visible in the iconography of their clinics. (3)

The two services also differed in the quality of the
care which they provided. This was not so much a question
of technical expertise as of organization. So far as
could be ascertained, there were few significant differences in the technical experience of the staff or the
quality of their work, although the American children's
hospital, as one of the centres of excellence in the
United States, offered more advanced orthopaedic care.
Many of the Scottish doctors had worked for a time in
hospitals in the United States and, although there was
not a reverse flow of similar proportions (only one of
the American doctors having worked in Britain), the
research of some of the Scottish doctors was known and
esteemed by their American equivalents.

If the differences in technical competence were relatively minor there were still significant differences in
the coherence, continuity and distribution of care between
the two services. In the American system patients were
not necessarily attached to any one practitioner and might
receive treatment for the same condition from a variety of
individual doctors, clinics and hospitals. Moreover,
there was no linked record system between these different
agents and agencies. The hospital only sent routine
reports on what they had done when a private practitioner
had referred a patient, while not all such practitioners
gave their records to hospital staff. Doctors at one city
hospital complained that private obstetricians sometimes
delivered a baby at the hospital and then left, taking the
records with them. By contrast in the Scottish system,
not only was each patient registered with one general
practitioner through whom both local authority doctors and
hospital specialists worked, but there were systematic
procedures for the exchange of essential information. The
local health authority was, for example, routinely sent
the discharge notes of all the babies who had been kept in
the Special Nursery and it maintained At Risk and Handicap
registers drawn both from their own staff's work and from
the hospital records. (4)

The systems also differed in the continuity of care
offered by the hospital service. Given the large turnover
of junior staff, both the American and Scottish hospitals
faced problems here; but the Scottish hospital made much
more systematic attempts to provide continuity of care for
at least some patients. Certain clinics, the special
clinics, were run just by one doctor, while in the general
clinics, the doctor in charge, normally a consultant,

tended to reserve the more long-term cases for himself. Moreover, it was hospital policy to continue to see many of the more severely handicapped cases long after it was medically necessary to do so. Many retarded children were, for instance, seen at six-monthly and then yearly intervals. In most of the American hospital clinics, such continuity of care was not so readily available for any except the wealthy, though some doctors made an exception with the occasional patient.

The overall coverage of the two systems also differed. In the American system, many fell through the net or were excluded, and no one organization had any responsibility for the entire community. In contrast to this, in the Scottish medical system there was not only a doctor allocated to every patient but, as has been noted, certain services were pressed on clients regardless of whether they had asked for them. As a result medical care was more generally spread throughout the population and some impairments in children were spotted much earlier than in the American system. This emphasis on the health of the total population was reflected even in the kinds of research done by some of the Scottish doctors. Just as there were great efforts to ensure that some services reached the total population, so too the funnelling of every patient into just the one agency meant that research into the characteristics of the total population was a relatively easy as well as a necessary task.

Finally, it may be noted that the different methods of financing health care affected not just the distribution of service but the mechanics of consultation. In the Scottish settings, since anyone was financially eligible and the transaction itself was not a unit of account, patients simply checked in at the appointments desk, had their consultation and left. By contrast, to attend an American clinic was a complex procedure in which one's financial as well as medical health was examined in detail. The American doctors did not deal directly with finance themselves, but such concerns permeated their work. The hospital social workers spent most of their time on financial matters and the doctors were obliged to consider how far any proposed action was covered by a particular insurance policy or state scheme.

Despite these considerable differences in the mode of organization, there were nevertheless some important similarities between the two systems. In both, specialist paediatrics was a recent creation. In the Scottish city there had been no full-time professor before the War, the chair being held part-time by a general practitioner. Similarly, the chief paediatrician at the American

children's hospital had fifteen years previously been the
sole paediatrician on staff, and then only as a joint
appointment with the main city hospital. Despite these
recent origins, the discipline had undergone tremendous
changes. Whereas the post-War battle had been to get
general paediatrics recognized as a proper medical
subject, the discipline was now fragmenting into a series
of specialisms and at the hospital level at least had
become increasingly research-oriented. So quickly had
this change occurred that one of the older Scottish staff
referred to himself as 'the first and last paediatrician'.
     There were also strong similarities as regards sexual
and professional stratification. In both services the
more presigious occupations were filled almost entirely
by men. All the staff doctors in the American children's
hospital were men, as were all the paediatricians in the
Scottish hospital at Consultant or Senior Registrar level,
with only one exception. On the other hand, all the
therapists and nurses in both institutions were women, as
were all the doctors that were observed in both the
Scottish local authority clinics and the American city
children's clinics. The social status of doctors was also
similar. There was a greater surface informality in the
American hospital - at least downwards - in that doctors
commonly called therapists and social workers by their
Christian names, a practice not normally observed in the
Scottish settings. It was also true that some therapists
and nurses had achieved a more specialist status in the
American hospital. Nevertheless in certain fundamental
ways they remained firmly under doctors' control, just as
in the Scottish hospital. Therapists, for example, could
obtain patients only through a doctor's referral, and
overall charge of the American therapy departments was
vested in a doctor.
     In both systems, hospitals depended heavily on trainee
labour. In both the children's hospitals the majority of
doctors held only temporary posts and were undergoing some
kind of training or aiming at some qualification. Indeed,
many of the junior doctors would eventually leave hospital
medicine altogether. Thus a great deal of work was done
under supervision, sometimes real, sometimes nominal.
     Despite this similarity there were also some important
differences here. Scottish medical students began
practising medicine two years later than their American
equivalents and also finished their training at a rather
later stage. Moreover, in the American hospital there was
no equivalent of the Senior Registrar level, that is of
doctors in their middle to late thirties. These Senior
Registrars formed an important resource in the Scottish

hospitals, situated as they were between the permanent staff and the relatively untrained junior staff, the registrars and housemen, who were the equivalent of the American interns and residents. This greater use of untrained staff in the American hospital may account for the wider range of questions and tests that were asked of and given to new patients there, as compared with the more focussed proceedings in the Scottish hospital. However, here as elsewhere, some may also discern financial motives (Janeway, 1974).

Keeping this rather crude summary of the two systems in mind, we may consider the particular settings that were studied and the types of case that were seen.

THE SCOTTISH CLINICS

In this, the major part of the study, nine different types of setting were observed, the bulk of them in the children's hospital. All of the clinics were run either by paediatricians or by therapists and, since some of the hospital doctors also taught in the local medical school, their students formed an audience in several of the settings. I shall consider each locale in turn.

The neurological clinic (children's hospital)

This was a special clinic run by a senior registrar. It had been created to give more time to handicapping conditions, and the cases seen here included cerebral palsy, epilepsy, breath-holding attacks, spina bifida, general retardation, muscular dystrophy, storage diseases, speech delay, speech problems, dwarfism and 'autism'. Certain important handicapping conditions were not seen at this clinic; for example, Down's syndrome (mongolism) and cystic fibrosis. The time actually spent with patients varied widely. Return patients where everything was under control, as in some epilepsy cases, might get only three minutes. Conversely, the most serious and complex chronic cases could take up to an hour, if a new case, or half an hour as a repeat.

This setting was observed for a three-year period, 113 clinics being attended in all. During this time, two doctors, Dr I and Dr J, ran the clinic, one doctor being observed in 82 clinics, the other doctor in 31. In all, 218 different children were observed in a total of 517 consultations.

The general medical clinics (children's hospital)

Each consultant paediatrician ran a general clinic which
took cases from across the whole range of paediatric work.
These included the standard child fare of chest complaints, allergies, urine infections in girls, hyperac-
tivity, headaches, 'failure to thrive', convulsions,
enuresis/encopresis, abdominal migraine/growing pains,
and examination for adoption, as well as a variety of
other problems such as congenital deformities, handicap,
metabolic disorders, rickets, worms, and various odd and
anomalous conditions. The clinics of two consultants,
Dr G and Dr H, were observed, one on six occasions and
with 51 cases, and the other on three occasions and with
16 cases. The average time spent by the first doctor on
new cases was eleven minutes, and on old cases six
minutes, though there was wide variation in the time
spent on individual cases. Such figures are impossible
to calculate for the second doctor, since he ran his
consultations in a different way. These clinics were the
main centre for outpatient teaching and training in paediatrics. Each consultant therefore worked with assistants,
often a registrar who saw cases in side-rooms, as well as
with an audience of medical students.

Physiotherapy (children's hospital)

This was a long-established department with three staff
and attached students, which took a wide variety of cases
of physical handicap on an outpatient basis. These were
seen weekly or fortnightly for half an hour at a time.
Inpatients were also treated, some on a daily basis. In
all, 29 cases and 59 treatment sessions were observed
here.

Occupational therapy (children's hospital)

This was a new department with two staff. Like physiotherapy it did both in- and outpatient work with handicapped children, but it also took some psychiatric cases;
27 cases were observed on 58 occasions.

The orthoptic clinic (children's hospital)

This clinic worked closely with the department of ophthal-
mology and was mainly involved in the treatment of squint.

It was staffed by one therapist, and 29 cases were seen at
seven sessions. These lasted an average of fifteen
minutes. This was the only one of the Scottish therapy
departments in which parents stayed during treatment.

Paediatric ward-rounds (maternity hospital)

All babies received a standard examination from a paediatrician at between 12 and 24 hours after birth. They
were then checked briefly every day. There were no home
confinements in the city, all births taking place in
either the maternity hospital or in one of the various
small maternity 'homes'. Mothers and babies in the
hospital were either at risk in some way, though normally
only very marginally so, or else medical staff themselves.·
Babies were normally kept by the mother's bedside and most
beds were on open or Nightingale wards, though there were
a variety of side-rooms which contained from one to five
beds. The ward-round was also an important vehicle for
training medical and nursing students. Four such rounds
were observed, in which 21 standard examinations were seen
and 154 other brief consultations. The ward-round was the
principal responsibility of one doctor, Dr K, though
another doctor was observed with a few babies.

Special nursery ward-round (maternity hospital)

Newborn babies who were in any way problematic were
admitted to the Special Nursery. Some babies were kept
in overnight if they appeared 'jittery', while other more
serious cases might spend several weeks there. At the
time of the study roughly 40 babies were in the nursery
at any one time. There was a daily ward-round by paediatric staff, which lasted about an hour and on which only
the more serious cases were dealt with in detail. Six
ward-rounds were observed over a period of a fortnight.

Special nursery follow-up clinic (maternity hospital)

All the children admitted to the Special Nursery were seen
at the follow-up clinic at the ages of 10 and 18 months,
although the more problematic cases might be seen both
earlier and more often. The clinic was staffed by a
paediatric senior registrar, Dr F, who carried out a brief
assessment of the child, the cases lasting between five
and ten minutes. Most children were discharged. Just one

doctor was seen here over four clinics and 27 cases.   This
clinic was also an important centre for teaching.   Observation at this and the general medical clinics was normally limited to occasions when only a few students were
present.

Local authority well-baby clinics

The health department of the city authorities ran baby
clinics located throughout the city and staffed by their
own doctors.   Any mother could bring her baby to such a
clinic as an alternative to visiting her general practitioner.   These clinics also carried out regular weighing
and immunization of babies.   In addition there was a
screening programme providing developmental assessment at
6 and 12 months for the entire age-group in the city.   An
average of four such assessments was scheduled for each
session of the clinic.   Five doctors, Dr A, Dr B, Dr C,
Dr D and Dr E, were observed in seven different locations,
and in these 18 clinic sessions and 112 consultations were
observed.

THE AMERICAN STUDY

The data in this study were far less extensive, although
a roughly comparable range of locales was observed.

The children's hospital

This was a private foundation and had originally served
'crippled children' only.   It now had a paediatric wing
where a wide variety of conditions was seen.   Two main
types of clinic were observed.   The first of these was
somewhat similar to those in the Scottish city and included neurological, developmental and general paediatric
clinics.   In all, five clinics of this type were visited
and a total of 12 sessions and 22 consultations observed,
though this latter figure relates only to cases where all
or a majority of the total consultation was seen.   Four
hospital staff doctors, Dr O, Dr P, Dr Q, Dr T, and five
junior doctors - interns and residents - were involved in
these cases.   In the second type of clinic, the 'amphitheatre clinic', a great many specialities were simultaneously involved.   All the other settings were based on the
principle of one clinic, one speciality.   In amphitheatre
clinics, which handled multiply-handicapping conditions

such as cerebral palsy and spina bifida, all the specialists deemed relevant attended. A total of four amphitheatre clinics, involving 18 consultations, were
observed. The work of three therapy departments (occupational, speech and physiotherapy) was also briefly seen,
with the observation of four sessions in all.

The city children's clinic

The city authorities ran a children's clinic catering for
children up to school age. It was lavishly equipped and
considered to be better than many such clinics in comparable cities. Since most of its clientele did not have a
general practitioner of their own, the clinic was the main
medical service for the children of the poor. There was
no total population screening programme. For those who
did turn up (and there was apparently a low attendance
rate), there was a set programme of assessment and immunization with six checks during the first year of a
baby's life and once a year after that till school age.
This clinic was attended over a two-day period, and four
doctors (including Dr S) and approximately 30 cases were
observed.

The state clinics

The state health department licensed city-run clinics and
provided certain specialist services for the poor in areas
where these were not available from other institutions.
Thus, although its headquarters were in the same city as
the children's hospital it ran no clinics there. Two
state clinics were visited in other cities, both sited in
rooms provided by a local hospital. One of these was run
by the 'Crippled Children's Service', while the other was
a developmental clinic which, like its counterpart in the
American children's hospital, included psychiatric as well
as paediatric aspects of development, a conjunction not
found in the Scottish clinics. In the state developmental
clinic one doctor, Dr R, and two cases were observed,
while in the Crippled Children's clinic, eight cases
attended by three doctors and one physiotherapist were
seen.

VARIATIONS WITHIN AND BETWEEN THE SETTINGS

The bare list of the clinics that were attended and the
numbers of cases that were seen gives little indication

of what went on there. To put some flesh on these dry
bones, I must describe, if only briefly, the kind of work
that went on, the people involved, and the various others
who were present.

Perhaps the most crucial feature of any consultation
was the type of condition presented by the patient and the
particular stage in its medical treatment at which the
consultation occurred. (5) Conditions may be distinguished along a number of dimensions as regards the medical
work which they entail. They differ widely as to the ease
with which they may be diagnosed; the extent to which the
doctor is reliant upon patients or parents for information; their seriousness; the ease with which they can
be treated; the length of time which treatment, if any,
may take; the accuracy with which their prognosis can be
foretold; the extent to which patients, parents or others
are in some way the 'cause' of the condition; the degree
to which treatment involves other departments and
services; and the extent to which staff are dependent on
patients' or parents' co-operation in their treatment.

Different cases combine these matters in different
ways. At one extreme in this study there was a case of
worms, where the diagnosis was immediate and drug therapy
was simple, quick and effective. At the other extreme
stood conditions like cerebral palsy. In its most severe
form, therapy was non-existent; aetiology, diagnosis and
prognosis might all be uncertain; a whole range of
medical and social services might be involved; and the
potential effects, both on the child and on its family,
were of the most appalling magnitude. In between these
polar types there were all manner of possible variations.

A second important variation in medical work concerns
the mode of referral. Where clients were self-referred
then a central task for both doctors and parents was the
presentation and discovery of a relevant medical problem.
By contrast, old patients or patients referred by another
doctor came with a problem that had already been certified
as relevant. Finally, there were some patients who in one
sense were not patients at all. In several settings
screening was a central medical activity. This was typically done to a formal agenda, unlike most other sorts of
medical investigation, and was not occasioned by a current
medical problem. It was a systematic search for problems
initiated by the profession rather than by the clientele,
and a search which normally proved fruitless, for most of
those screened were passed as normal.

Settings also differed widely in the extent to which
staff had a mandate for treatment or diagnosis. In some
Scottish settings (for example, the local authority

clinics and the special nursery follow-up clinic) doctors
had no such mandate;   their job was solely assessment and
diagnosis.   Where treatment was required the patients had
to be passed on to other clinics for, just as some clinics
specialized in diagnosis, others specialized in treatment.
At the extreme here were the therapy clinics where
diagnosis was the principal responsibility of the doctor,
and therapists merely elaborated on the initial diagnosis
for the purposes of treatment.   (This at least was the
form of the thing if not always the practice.)
    Since clinics differed systematically in their mix of
conditions, their referral procedures and their mandate,
their atmosphere showed significant variation (Davis and
Strong, 1976b).   For example, although screening could
potentially threaten the normality of any child, this had
most effect in the special nursery follow-up clinic, since·
all the children there had been defined as problematic at
birth.   By contrast, in the American city and Scottish
local authority clinics, screening was a routine and
normally jolly affair.   Clinics also showed systematic
differences in the extent to which doctors, patients and
parents could get to know each other.   In those clinics
where a high proportion of children were discharged, as
in the screening clinics or the general paediatric
clinics, everything was geared to a rapid turnover of
clientele.   Others by contrast, like the neurological
clinic, saw a much smaller number of patients, more intensively and over a longer period of time.
    A further important source of variation lay in the kind
of adult representative who accompanied a child.   Normally
this was the mother, and it was also normal for the mother
to be the child's sole representative.   This occurred in
roughly 900 of the consultations.   In all, only 67 couples
were observed in a total of 107 occasions.   Only 14
fathers were seen alone with a child.   Grandmothers were
a slightly more frequent representative;   they accompanied
18 different children at a total of 30 consultations.
Apart from this, mothers were accompanied by grandmothers
on five occasions, and by grandfathers on another three
occasions.   Many more fathers and grandparents accompanied
mother and child to the clinic but did not actually enter
the consulting room.   Apart from relatives, foster-parents
and social workers might also act as representatives for a
child;   17 foster-mothers were observed on 25 different
occasions, and house-mothers from local children's homes
brought children on another 25 occasions.   Sometimes
social workers also accompanied a child, though never by
themselves.   They were present overall at 12 consultations.

The extent to which both parents rather than just
mothers were present varied significantly according to
the severity of the child's condition.   Thus the Scottish
neurological clinic had by far the highest proportion of
cases in which both parents came with the child.   Out of
218 cases that were observed here, 52 (26 per cent) had
both parents present in at least one consultation.   In
the total number of consultations (518) a slightly smaller
proportion of couples were present (96 or 19 per cent).
By contrast, in the eight Scottish general medical clinics
there were only four couples present in 67 consultations
(6 per cent of the total).   Even this might be considered
relatively high, for not one couple attended any of the
112 Scottish local authority clinic consultations or
brought along their child to any of the Scottish therapy
sessions.   The same was also true of the American city
children's clinic.   Although insufficient numbers of cases
were observed in any one American hospital clinic to
permit such generalization, six out of the total of 55
cases seen in the hospital were accompanied by both of
their parents (11 per cent).   In both hospitals middle-
class children were more likely to be accompanied by both
their parents than working-class children, as were
children who lived some distance away compared with those
resident in the city.

Some clinics also differed in the class and ethnic
background of the parents.   In the Scottish clinics,
almost all patients belonged to the same ethnic group;
for there were no immigrant minorities in the city of any
size, unless English and American residents count as such.
Moreover there was only one Scottish setting, the local
authority clinics, in which there was any distinct class
bias in the nature of the clientele at any one clinic –
a product of the residential location of the different
clinics.   In contrast, certain of the American services
were specifically for the poor;   and even within the
children's hospital, private patients were seen by some,
though not all, doctors in their own room rather than in
the general clinics.   Further, the American city had a
large black and Puerto Rican population, with both groups
living largely in semi-ghetto conditions.   The Puerto
Ricans in particular formed a distinct cultural minority
and many had little grasp of English.

Having discussed the kinds of adult who accompanied
children, we may now consider the staff.   At the same time
I shall also comment on the rooms in which the consultations took place, for the kind of staff who were present
strongly influenced the design of the setting.   At one
extreme were some of the American private consultations

and the Scottish local authority clinics. In both of
these each child and parent was seen by one doctor in a
large room with no one else present, apart from the
researcher. The doctor sat behind a desk and patients
were shown in one by one as their turn came. At the
opposite end of the spectrum there were a variety of
settings in which consultations took place in the presence
of many other people, sometimes patients, sometimes staff,
sometimes both, some of whom had rights to intervene in
the action. For instance, in some of the therapy departments several children were treated at the same time
by different therapists in just the one large room.

In the amphitheatre clinics in the American hospital,
consultations took place on a floodlit stage in front of
a large audience of doctors, therapists, nurses, social
workers, interns and residents, who sat in tiered seats
in semi-darkness. Although one doctor typically controlled the occasion, there might be two or three staff on the
stage all playing a part. Members of the audience might
also join in: by calling out comments and questions, by
being asked their opinions, or by coming on to the stage
themselves.

In the paediatric ward-round at the Scottish maternity
hospital the majority of mothers were in large Nightingale
wards and the doctor was often accompanied by a group of
medical students or trainee nurses. Doctors conversed
with the mothers at the bedside, normally without the use
of screens, so that most of what happened was both audible
and visible to the other mothers in the ward. Such rounds
were watched with keen interest by this audience, who
joined in on occasion with jokes and comments.

In between these extremes there were many consultations
which took place in a single room, but where there was an
audience of nurses and students of variable size. In the
Scottish children's hospital, general paediatric clinics
were located in a suite of three rooms. In the middle and
larger room the consultant sat behind a wide desk. To one
side of this desk there were chairs placed for the child
and family, to the other side there were one or more rows
of chairs for medical students, of whom up to seven or
eight might be present during term. In the side-rooms,
which were much smaller in size, the junior doctors saw
their patients. In some instances these doctors consulted
with the senior doctor present before finishing a case.
Patients were booked for different times in the afternoon
and waited upon their arrival in a special area at the far
end of a corridor. When their turn came they were shown
into the appropriate room by nursing staff, who also
showed them out when their appointment had finished. The

Scottish neurological clinic was also based on such a
suite of rooms, but the doctor occupied only the large
room and the audience was far smaller. A nurse was
usually present during the consultations, as was a
secretary for a planned assessment centre. Students
attended on occasion; but here as elsewhere in the
Scottish hospital they played a passive role in the
consultations. Only on the ward-round at the maternity
hospital did they play any active part in the examination
of the patients.

By contrast, in the American children's hospital the
outpatient or ambulatory clinic consisted of a long
corridor on which were located a dozen small, windowless
cubicles, each with an examination couch and two chairs.
In the middle and on one side of the corridor there was
a large room out of which all the doctors and students
worked. This room contained all the 'files' or 'charts'
of the clinic cases, as well as chairs, coffee and a bank
of phones for dictating notes. This served as a private
room for the discussion of cases. There was no door on
this room and although there were doors on the cubicles
these were kept open most of the time, as they were
claustrophobic when kept shut. All the patients were
booked for the same time, and those who arrived first
were shown immediately into the vacant cubicles. The rest
of the patients and their parents waited in easy chairs at
the far end of the corridor. Interns and residents
'worked up' the patients in the cubicles and then left to
consult with their 'chief'. Since a chief might have to
advise up to six or seven of the more junior doctors,
though the latter gave considerable help to each other,
the patients often had to wait for considerable periods
of time. The layout and practice of the American city
children's clinic was very similar, except that here it
was nurses, not interns and residents, who did the work-
up. In summary, the difference between the two outpatient
departments was that in the Scottish hospitals the patient
was brought to the doctor, whereas in the American hospitals the doctor came to the patient.

Some consideration must be given to the activities of
the nursing staff in these various settings, for they had
an important facilitative role. Whereas therapists worked
by themselves, doctors in the hospital clinics were aided
by nurses who performed a variety of minor but important
tasks. One job common to all settings was that of gate-
keeper. Nurses regulated the flow of patients to the
doctor and monitored them in the waiting area. They
checked appointments against lists, told doctors when
patients had arrived, warned them when parents had got

fed up with waiting, and accompanied patients when they
left. They also handled incoming phone calls, telephoned
other departments, fixed admissions, checked on patients
who were attending other clinics, and handled relations
with the appointments and records staff. They might also
regulate visitors to the clinic, such as other doctors,
students and researchers.

Nurses might also play an important role in the prepa-
ration and examination of patients. They weighed and
measured children, took urine samples, checked that the
records were available, took patients to X-ray, calmed
children during examination, and generally helped out in
any of a great number of problems that might arise. They
sometimes, for example, stepped in to clear up a misunderstanding between doctor and patient. These duties were
taken rather further in the American settings. In the
ambulatory clinics at the hospital, the nurses performed
various psychological tests, and in the city children's
clinic they did the entire work-up. In both systems they
also prepared each clinic for the day's work, generally
arriving before the doctors and reading through the
records to see what might be needed, and what eventuali-
ties might occur. They laid out the seating and trolleys
and saw that all the files were present.

Where there were several doctors working in a clinic,
nurses could have a crucial role in ordering the whole
occasion. In one of the Scottish general clinics this
role was taken by the consultant but in the other, as in
the American clinics, the nurse on duty took charge. She
reminded interns when they had left a patient sitting in
a cubicle for thirty minutes, advised the more junior
doctors on what cases they would find easy or interesting,
and generally made sure that things were running smoothly.

Although nurses had fewer medical responsibilities in
the Scottish clinics, they had by and large more say in
doctors' actual interaction with the patients. In the
American hospital the division of labour between juniors
and chiefs and the tiny space in the cubicles meant that
the American nurses, when they were not administering
tests or weighing patients, spent much of their time in
the duty room. Scottish nurses, however, spent long
periods in the same room with the doctor and their role
was more like that of a personal secretary. A skilled
nurse knew what each doctor liked and disliked. One
wanted his desk prepared just so, the telephone in exactly
this position and the files in that. Another did not mind
about his desk but had his own special arrangements about
how patients should be prepared. Each doctor had his own
set sequences of action and special signals to indicate

what was to be done. The nurse who knew these could move
swiftly to the doctor's aid almost before he had moved,
turning off the lights for an eye-examination or holding
a child during a physical. In such ways Scottish doctors
became heavily dependent on the nursing staff; and the
absence of a regular nurse was cursed by every doctor, for
things kept on going wrong and nothing was in its right
place: 'It just isn't the same when Staff's not here.'

Some nurses tried to aid doctors in yet another way.
They stood and talked in the corridor to old patients, and
commiserated with them when they had to wait a long time.
They chatted away as they prepared a child for the clinic
or guided parents to another part of the hospital. In
doing this they gleaned a good deal of background information about the parents and their lives. Such detail was
obviously of major interest to the nursing staff but
little use of it was made by doctors. Nurses often wished
to chat about a particularly striking case, to grieve,
enthuse, moan or gossip. Doctors rarely did, but pressed
on to the next case. In consequence nurses only occasionally reported what they had uncovered and then only when
the news was of the greatest relevance: that this mother
was an alcoholic, or so her grandfather had hinted; or
that that mother was very angry with the doctor as she
felt the drugs had caused a recent bout of vomiting.

A MORAL

The main point of this rapid tour is this: here was a
considerable variety of clinics - set in two very different kinds of medical system, one of which encompassed a
great range of types of practice - and to these clinics
came all kinds and conditions of patients and parents;
yet, as I have argued and as I shall go on to demonstrate,
the ceremonial order of the consultations was remarkably
invariant. To repeat my earlier assertion, not only were
there institutionalized role formats, but their number was
severely limited and of these, one - the bureaucratic
format - was to be found in universal though not sole use
in every type of setting observed in the study. In each
clinic, most consultations were framed by the bureaucratic
format most of the time or, put another way, though they
met in all manner of circumstances, doctors and parents
routinely transcended the mundane particularities of their
meeting and invested themselves and their relationship
with much the same ritual form.

Why this one form was chosen rather than any other is
a question which must be left to the end of this mono-

graph. For the moment I shall concentrate on its description; a task which requires several chapters, for
the rules on which it was based, though relatively simple,
required some care in their enactment.

Before I begin, two general points should be borne in
mind. Both concern the procedures used by the participants to rise above the actual circumstance of their
meeting.

First, even where a rule characterized only one of the
parties, its creation and maintenance were the work of
both staff and parents: the bureaucratic format was a
collaborative effort. Second, although there were a
variety of rules within the format all were established
by the same fundamental procedure, that of avoidance.
Rules were maintained by ignoring those matters which they
could not cover. This device, or as Goffman (1961) has
termed it, the 'rule of irrelevance', is the basic
procedure used to sustain any encounter, wherever it may
occur. For present purposes in interaction, any features
of the setting that do not fit, any qualities of the
participants, any emotions or attitudes and any involvements in other action: all these, if they form no
part of the current order, are treated as irrelevant. We
make a world and behave, for the moment, as if we could
not see the wider worlds from which it was made and in
which it is situated. Children when they play a game may
turn themselves into soldiers, old clothes into uniforms,
and chairs and tables into forts. Similar, if less
readily visible transformations occur in any adult
encounter.

This magic, if I can use the term for so routine a
human accomplishment, is not always made with ease. There
are some things which will not disappear if we merely shut
our eyes, but require a little work if they are to vanish.
My account of each rule is therefore in two main parts.
Where the trick was pulled with ease, the rule itself was
invisible. In consequence, the demonstration of its
existence requires a detailed comparison with other
formats in which a different principle held sway. By
contrast, where active nullification was required, the
work that was necessary to render other matters irrelevant
made the operation of the rule and thus the rule itself at
least partially apparent.

3 Natural parenthood

Of the various rules which made up the bureaucratic format
the first which I shall examine concerns the identity
ascribed to parents. As we shall see, what parents were
actually like: whether they really loved a child or not;
the degree of competence with which they cared for it;
the responsibility which they themselves might bear for a
child's condition - none of these things were at issue, at
least on the surface, and none of them affected the
idealized image which parents were granted.

Thus, although children were represented by others, all
was for the best, since their representatives were very
special sorts of people. Matters could hardly be otherwise, for the qualities ascribed to parents were seen as
entirely natural in origin; they went with the job.
Every mother, just because she was a mother, was an ideal
mother, someone who naturally wanted and loved her
children and cared for them with a wholly natural competence. (1) Likewise, every mother made an ideal representative. Children might not know how to fend for themselves in medical consultations; but there was little to
fear, for their mothers were honest, intelligent, reliable
and impartial; or so the story ran.

Not only were mothers possessed of these admirable
qualities; but their worth was such that their presence
alone, along with the child, was a sufficient condition
for a proper consultation to take place. On only a
handful of occasions, all involving the breaking of bad
news, were both parents requested to attend; and even
here this request was by no means typical.

If the mother could not be present, though as we have
seen she normally was, then either the father or a
grandparent would do; but both were normally treated as
substitutes for the real thing. Even so they too were
idealized in their own fashion and ascribed a suitable
measure of virtues.

Given the ideal nature ascribed to mothers and, as will
be seen in the next two chapters, the equivalent idealization of staff's competence and motivation, medical
consultations within the bureaucratic format were extremely polite affairs. Many formal courtesies were paid to
parents, questions were asked in a mild tone of voice, and
considerable effort was normally made to respect their
feelings. Staff made many apologies: for keeping parents
waiting; for delays in getting test results; for
misunderstandings; or for making mothers repeat stories
which they had already told before. In general there was
an air of some gentility, harsh or bad language was
avoided, and the best rather than the worst was overtly
assumed about those present. There was, of course, some
variation in these matters; particular staff on particular occasions were more or less courteous, and sometimes
their impatience or irritation were only barely concealed.
Nevertheless the predominant tenor of the proceedings was
politeness.

The mechanisms through which parents were idealized
form the main body of this chapter. However, before I go
on to describe these it may be useful to begin in quite
another way: by making a comparison with a separate
format in which mothers were vilified rather than sancti-
fied. And to do this I must first describe the nature of
idealization and its counterpart a little more closely.

CHARACTER WORK AND THE CHARITY FORMAT

Identity is the central topic on which any ceremonial
order legislates, and moral status is a fundamental part
of that identity. But since the ceremonial order is a
matter of outward show, the moral order which it creates
is regularly threatened by the actual facts of the case
and by the incidents and upsets that occur in any form of
human intercourse. In consequence, the parties to an
encounter are presented with a series of constant
challenges, either actual or potential, which threaten
their moral worth or that of their fellow-participants.
The ways in which such challenges are handled may be
called 'moral work' (Strong and Davis, 1978), and within
this we may distinguish two main types of response. The
first, which Goffman (1972) has termed 'face-work', is a
kind of running repair: the ascribed identity and moral
status of the individual is treated as the true reality
and any discrepancies between the two are simply glossed
over.

There is another type of moral work, one which may be

called 'character-work'. Unlike face-work this is only
rarely used in encounters, for it does not concern the
maintenance of a smooth surface appearance but involves
the uncovering of a person's moral essence, a rather more
tricky endeavour. That essence, or the everyday concept
of character, refers to an assumed moral core, inherent
within individuals and transcending any particular social
occasion. Character on this account is what people
'really' are underneath it all. Whereas face-work
attempts to preserve the ideal image that a person may
present in any one encounter, character-work seeks to go
behind this and explore the reality. Face-work is microscopic in focus and serves to smooth the present, while
character-work is more explicitly concerned with future
behaviour and the effects of the individual on society at
large.

Since character-work is exploratory, it varies according to what is uncovered and may take one of two forms
when wrong-doing is revealed. In the first of these,
which may be termed 'ameliorative', the procedures are
those of criticism and exhortation to reform. In the
second and stronger type - 'reconstitutive' work - such
measures are too late and there is nothing left but to
proclaim the individual's fundamental immorality. (2)

Having made all these distinctions we can now put them
to some use in considering the 'charity format', a mode
whose nature was quite separate from the smooth politeness
of the bureaucratic form. The charity format was not at
all common; indeed only one doctor in the entire study
was observed to use it. (3) Nevertheless, through
studying it we may learn much about what was avoided
elsewhere.

Whereas face-work was the staple diet of the bureaucratic format, character-work was the standard fare in
the charity mode. The doctor who used it, a doctor in
the clinic run by the American city, distinguished three
types of moral character in mothers. (4) First there were
the penitent and eager to learn. Second, there were those
who might seem overtly penitent but whose capacity or
willingness to make amends was in some doubt. Finally,
there were the impenitent or those of revealed bad
character. In the 15 consultations all but two mothers
were identified as being of the second, rather dubious
type, for the standards set to enter the first category
were those of the doctor herself. To count as moral and
competent and to be treated as such, mothers had to do
exactly what she would have done; and she was middle-
class, white and medically trained, whereas the mothers
were poor and mostly black or Puerto Rican.

The only mother with whom the doctor enjoyed an easy relationship was a young white woman of serious demeanour who engaged in self-criticism. She described how she fed the child, mentioned what she had read about feeding and asked for the doctor's advice in this matter. In all, she enacted the role of a humble but keen medical student. In return the doctor provided her with reassurance and a mass of technical information. But other mothers did not formally ask her advice, nor did they mention any books or articles they had read and thus demonstrate their concern. They were therefore subjected to forceful interrogation, which undercut any of their claims to competence as a mother. Here, for example, is an excerpt from a case in which the presenting problem was nappy rash. All the doctor's remarks were made in a most aggressive fashion:

Dr S: What do you wash her nappies in?
Mother: Ivory Snow.
Dr S: Why do you use Ivory Snow?
Mother: Well, it's supposed to make the nappies softer
        than other washing powders.
Dr S: How do you know Ivory Snow makes nappies softer?
Mother: (shrugs awkwardly) Well, um ... (she mumbles
        something about her mother and advertisements).
Dr S: You don't want to believe everything you see in
      the adverts. It's a business. That's *their*
      business. *Your* business is your baby.

The doctor then explained that nappy rash was due to ammonia in the urine and that Ivory Snow was too weak. The mother should therefore use an ordinary washing powder.

Mother: I do put vinegar in it.
Dr S: (in amazed tone) Why do you do that?
Mother: Well, I was told.
Dr S: Who told you?
Mother: Well, my mother did.
Dr S: What difference does it make?
Mother: Well, she said ... I thought it ...
Dr S: It doesn't do any good at all.

The doctor then gave an explanation of the chemistry involved.
Since the doctor held that the only rational criteria for behaviour were her own, those who behaved in a different fashion were deemed irrational, and ignorance was seen as a lack of love towards the child and even, on some

occasions, as proof of hatred: feeding a two-and-a-half-month baby on solid food was characterized as a 'hostile' action.

Although the doctor denounced many mothers in private, her normal strategy was ameliorative. She urged mothers to repent and was often most rude, but overtly she still had hopes of reform. In one case matters took a different turn; and since the outcome was so exceptional it is worth considering in some detail. The issue on which everything revolved was demeanour. In criminal pro-ceedings the character assigned to the guilty person often rests on the agent's decision as to whether due contrition has been demonstrated (Piliavin and Briar, 1964). In this one case the mother, an unmarried black woman, laughed when describing one of her child's problems, and the doctor instantly switched from amelio-rative to reconstitutive work:

> Dr S: Are there any other problems?
> Mother: Well, he chews cigarette ends ... (laughs)....
>   It's very difficult to stop him.
> Dr S: Why are you laughing? Do you think it's funny?
> Mother: No, I don't think it's funny.
> Dr S: Well, why did you laugh then; do you always
>   laugh at this?

Reconstitutive work was quite different from that used with other parents. Apart from calling the mother to account for her demeanour, something that was not done elsewhere - parents were normally given great latitude here - the doctor repeatedly tried to expose contra-dictions in the mother's story and show that she was lying. In all the other cases in this study there was an overt assumption that mothers were telling the truth. Contradictions were treated as mistakes or surface ob-scurities and normally went unremarked. But here they were explicitly sought out in order to prove that the mother was truly a bad character. For example:

> Dr S: So you entirely ignore it when he starts chewing
>   cigarettes?
> Mother: No, I don't.
> Dr S: Well, why did you say you did?
> Mother: I didn't.

Apart from trying to prove the mother a liar, the doctor also mocked her intelligence. Whereas in other cases this was never openly questioned by staff, here the doctor jeered at things that the mother had forgotten, and criti-cized her use of English. For example:

> Mother: It looks so stupid when you see a fine-looking
>   man with his feet turned in like that. I don't
>   want my baby growing up like that. (The child
>   has turned-in feet.)
> Dr S: What do you mean by stupid? Do you think your
>   brains are in your feet?

Finally, the doctor engaged in a wide-ranging search to
find other failings in the mother. Unlike her practice in
other cases she did not concentrate on merely the one
problem and its reform, but treated the initial crime as
symptomatic of a much wider range of abuses. Just as
face-work could prove that a mother was entirely good, so
reconstitutive work could demonstrate her complete iniqui-
ty; for it is characteristic of our treatment of those
found to be unrepentantly deviant that emphasis is placed,
not upon the initial sin, but upon the corrupted character
of which the present sin is merely a symptom. Apart from
quizzing the mother about her attempts to stop the child
chewing cigarettes, the doctor interrogated her for
several minutes about where she kept poisons in the house,
and asked detailed questions concerning the child's care
and the mother's marital and financial status, all of
which were put in a hostile and sceptical fashion; her
aim being to prove the mother uncaring, promiscuous, work-
shy and sponging off the state.

NATURAL MOTHERHOOD

This sketch of the procedures used in the charity format
can also tell us much about the bureaucratic mode. For
what was raised in one form had to be avoided in the
other. The rule that every mother was a good mother meant
the systematic exclusion of all those things that were
explicitly raised when character-work was done. In the
bureaucratic format doctors had to strive to use a polite
rather than an aggressive tone; to ignore inconsisten-
cies; to avoid open condemnation; and to stick to the
matter in hand rather than search for fault upon fault.
And they had to do this whatever their actual feelings
about the circumstance of the case.

But staff were also involved in more positive work, for
a mother's good character could not always be guaranteed
through passing some things by in silence. Certain disreputable topics necessarily intruded into the conversation and on some occasions doctors could not avoid
criticism of what mothers had done. Some regularly missed
appointments and others were highly incompetent. For some

conditions a mother might reasonably be held to be partially or even wholly responsible. In other cases mothers refused to accept the doctor's version of the child, and in yet others they were unable to cope with it, whereas all mothers were supposed to have this capacity. Some mothers lived disreputable lives and on occasion inquiry into these was medically unavoidable.

The wide variety of circumstances in which a more active face-work was necessary meant that doctors' tactics varied to suit these. For example, the paediatrician who did the ward-round at the Scottish maternity hospital called all mothers 'Mrs' regardless of their marital status. But this imposition was not always possible. On some occasions inquiry had to be made into private lives and, since the doctor could not know in advance what would be found, the mother's good character was often maintained by making no overt assumptions at all, by treating any household arrangement as a simple matter of fact:

Dr G: Is there anybody else in the house with you?
Mother: Well, my husband.

Despite this necessary variation in tactics, certain broad medical strategies may be discerned within the bureaucratic format. When criticism had to be done, doctors emphasized the spotless future rather than the murky past. Here, for instance, is a quotation from a Scottish local authority clinic in which a mother was interviewed about her grossly overweight baby, who at six months was covered in rolls of fat and weighed 20 pounds:

Dr B: And you feed him on Farex?
Mother: In the morning and evening.
Dr B: And porridge?
Mother: Aye.
Dr B: Does he get anything else for elevenses?
Mother: Just biscuits.
Dr B: How much porridge does he get?
Mother: Oh, nae much.
Dr B: How much does he get at lunch-time?
Mother: Oh, just mince and tatties.
Dr B: Do you give him anything in mid-afternoon?
Mother: No.
Dr B: And what does he get for his tea?
Mother: Oh, a boiled egg or a scrambled egg.
Dr B: And this is as well as milk?
Mother: Aye.
Dr B: Does he get anything else?
Mother: Aye.... (rest inaudible)

Dr B: Well, I think he's putting on a bit too much
weight.   Is he fatter than your other children?
Mother: Aye.
Dr B: If I were you I'd miss out the Farex and the
porridge at breakfast and the biscuit as well.
It's best to do this now because if children get
fat now then they tend to be fatter later on in
life.   He's supposed to be twice his birthweight
now and he's a good bit more than that, isn't he?
This is very important.   He's putting on a bit
too much weight.

If one contrasts this with the case of nappy rash discussed earlier, several important differences emerge.   Far
from being aggressive the doctor here posed her questions
in a neutral fashion, as if they were purely a matter of
form, while her advice at the end was given in a breezy
and non-pejorative manner.   At the same time, the seriousness of the problem and thus of the possible offence was
under-played.   It might be 'very important', but then he
was only putting on 'a bit too much weight'.   The most
crucial difference lay in the focus of the discussion.
The doctor who inquired about feeding asked solely about
what the mother did.   By contrast, although the other
mother's behaviour was mentioned - her use of Ivory Snow
and vinegar - the charity doctor's emphasis was upon the
beliefs that underlay those practices.   Since she indicated by her whole manner that these were incorrect, to
ask the mother persistently for the grounds for her action
was to ask her to make a fool of herself.   Indeed, to
conduct any detailed inquiry into the grounds for
someone's action is to imply that they have acted
incorrectly.   The reasons why we act as we do normally
go unspoken.   They are presumed to be obvious and in good
faith and are only revealed when others judge us, or might
do so.   The result of such inquiry in the American clinic
was that the mother became increasingly unwilling to
answer the questions, began to mumble and eventually broke
off in embarrassment.   By contrast, the matter-of-fact
inquiry into actions rather than beliefs meant that the
Scottish mother responded in a free and open fashion.
Further, when the doctor in this latter case delivered
her verdict this was done in a fashion that did not necessarily question the mother's competence.   The doctor
treated herself as an expert who knew things that the
mother did not, but the mother was not cast as a fool.
The doctor simply told the mother what the 'best' thing
to do was, that it was 'important', and that if she were
in the mother's place then this is what she would do:

'If I were you'. She presented the mother as agreeing
with the wisdom of what she had said: 'Isn't he?' Her
strategy was to spell out what she saw as the correct
policy and then to demonstrate that this was the sensible
thing that anyone would do, once they knew the facts. The
emphasis was not upon the mother's mistake but upon the
right thing to do in the future. The charity doctor
operated like a policeman for whom ignorance of the law
was no excuse. By conducting an interrogation about the
past she emphasized the mother's guilt. The Scottish
doctor emphasized the mother's future action which, it was
overtly assumed, would be correct now that she had learnt
what to do. Such a strategy allowed the mother to retain
her ideal character. Her competence did not lie in
knowing what was the best way of bringing up a healthy
baby, that was a matter for the doctor. It rested instead
on taking an active interest in her child's health and in
following good advice.

Even if mothers did not follow staff's instructions,
they could still retain their overt good character within
the bureaucratic format. Doctors did not press hard,
except where the most serious matters were at stake, and
even then they still used the same, future-oriented
strategy. The past was written off and parents once more
had a chance to prove themselves. This emerges most
clearly if we consider the one matter about which all
Scottish hospital staff got worked up: failure to attend.
The only basic demands made of mothers were that they
attend the clinic when asked to do so and, if this should
prove impossible, that they give prior warning. For a
mother to meet either of these conditions ensured her
treatment as entirely competent and moral, regardless of
any other circumstances. Part of the reason for this
priority lay in the appointments system. Since parents
were booked at particular times their non-arrival might
leave staff with nothing to do, a major irritant for those
with many other demands on their time. And, of course,
parents who did not appear not only failed the doctor but
they failed their children as well - patients who could
not attend on their own behalf.

It would therefore be no surprise if doctors' irritation or anger occasionally surfaced here. One mother,
for example, had missed three appointments; at the end
of the consultation at which she finally appeared, the
doctor commented with heavy sarcasm, 'Thank you very much
for bringing her to see us'. And yet what is truly re-
markable about this comment is its exceptional nature:
it was the most critical statement made to a mother in any
of the Scottish clinics. Other staff, and indeed this

same doctor on other occasions, behaved in a quite different fashion. They still treated non-attendance as a
serious matter, for they routinely asked mothers to
provide reasons why they had not come on a previous occasion. On this issue at least they dug up the past. But
they did so in a way which removed any overt implication
that this was a moral investigation. Not only did they
conduct their inquiry politely but, although they called
mothers to account, they commonly furnished them with good
excuses in doing so. 'Have you moved?' 'Did you lose
your appointment card?' 'Have you been ill?' 'Have there
been any problems with transport?' Questions such as
these both required a reason, and suggested that the
answer would indeed be reasonable. In this way, while
attention was drawn to a fault, the offence was indicated
to be a misdemeanour and the questioning in no way
threatened their overt good character.

By such means within the bureaucratic format staff
routinely transformed the possible crimes committed by
mothers into something that was readily compatible with
the ideal that every mother was supposed to be. They did
so by skirting around some issues; by minimizing their
offence; by providing them with good excuses; and finally by dismissing the past as of no account. In fact, such
was the commitment of doctors to the idealization of their
clientele that they attempted this even when they got no
support from the mothers themselves. So far I have made
no mention of the mothers' own cosmetic practices but left
the reader to assume that they co-operated readily with
staff in this regard. Normally this was indeed so. There
were however two exceptions. But even here the doctors
tried to demonstrate the mothers' good character and
competence. Since these two cases represent the greatest
test to which idealization was put, some space must be
devoted to them, though I shall examine only one in
detail.

In the first of these cases the mother was mentally
retarded, and this status was publicly if indirectly
displayed. To be retarded is to have grave doubts cast
on one's ability to represent or care for a child; and
in fact this mother was accompanied by a social worker
who treated her in many ways as if she too were a child.
She regularly intervened to correct the mother's account
and, when she did so, spoke about the mother as if she
were not there and able to speak for herself. The mother
acquiesced in all this quite willingly and showed no signs
of irritation or embarrassment at being interrupted or
discussed in this fashion. After each of her own remarks,
whether they were questions or replies, she gave a special

kind of grin, self-deprecating and self-consciously
childish, such as no other parent gave. This grin was
a constant and deliberate reminder to her audience that
she was formally defined as retarded. Its message was
that she was doing her best, that she was trying to be
helpful, but that she was retarded and not to be blamed
for any mistakes she might make.

The oddity of the mother's behaviour and of the
treatment she was accorded is summed up by the manner in
which new instructions about the dosage of a drug were
given and received. The mother listened to the instructions in a fashion unlike any other adult representative, her whole body overtly tensed in the most
extraordinary way and her eyes riveted upon the doctor.
The only comparison to be made is with the behaviour of
young children during testing, some of whom assumed the
same pose of totally committed and forceful concentration.
Just as such children would suddenly break off and
announce that they could no longer continue, so too this
mother, without any warning, blurted out that she could
not remember what the doctor had said. He therefore sat
beside her and, at the social worker's suggestion, gave
her written as well as verbal instructions, two procedures
that were never followed in other cases.

Although the doctor treated the mother in a special
way, what was equally striking was his consistent attempt
to define her as competent. When parents interrupted
their children's remarks the conversation normally stayed
with them and the child was excluded from then on. Here,
however, the doctor reverted to the mother each time with
only the slightest acknowledgment, if any, of most of the
social worker's comments. Even when the doctor wrote out
his instructions and discussed these with the social
worker, he still indicated his trust in the mother's
competence:

> Dr I: If James has just one fit then she (the mother)
> can still stop the phenobarbitone as he's likely
> to have one or two anyway. But if he has more,
> then she should immediately start James on the
> phenobarbitone again.
> Social Worker: How will she know if he has attacks?
> She may miss them.
> Dr I: (to mother) I don't think you miss them very
> easily, do you? Because you can tell by the way
> he breathes.
> Mother: Yes, he has funny breathing, yes.
> Dr I: And you sleep fairly close to him, don't you?
> Mother: Yes.

Dr I: (to social worker) So I don't think she would
      miss many.

Although this case was exceptional, it being the only
occasion on which a mother who was actually present at the
consultation was herself represented by another adult,
there are some interesting parallels with the problems
that might arise when both parents were present. For,
just as intervention by the social worker could undercut
the mother's story, so too one spouse might contradict
another. To take one example from many:

Dr J: How about his speech? Is that OK?
Mother: Yes, he uses a lot of words.
Dr J: When did this start?
Mother: Well, he's been saying 'Mammy' and 'Daddy' for
        a long time. And he's been saying more than
        this for quite ... (pause) ... Well ...
        (pause) ... this past two months he's been
        really chatting.
Dr J: For how long?
Mother: The past couple of months.
Father: Oh, it's been longer, surely?
Mother: No, he only said 'Mammy' and 'Daddy' before.
Father: No. You think about it. He used to say
        'Daddy's car' ... (he gives two further
        examples) ... He's been saying these for quite
        a long time.

Such conflict was resolved by the mother being given
priority – but at the same time this was done discreetly.
Staff did not ask parents to make their minds up, nor did
they come down too openly on the mother's side. Such
disagreements were treated as private quarrels in which
staff had no part to play. They became a sideshow, not
a part of the main action; and staff waited until they
were finished before resuming their questioning or discussion. The only comment that any doctor actually made
on these matters was to lean forward to a young girl, some
aspect of whom the parents were disputing at considerable
length, and remark, 'They're talking about you.'
    In the other case in which a doctor took an advocate
role on the mother's behalf despite her rejection of the
proffered ideal, the child was neglected (it had recurrent
scabies and a skin-rash) and had not been brought to the
clinic for some time for consideration of its severe
cerebral palsy. As in the previous case, the mother was
accompanied to the clinic, this time by a health visitor,
though she, unlike the social worker, did not actually

enter the consulting room. The good character of the
mother was nevertheless clearly in doubt, a possibility
that was reinforced by her demeanour. She remained sullen
and accusatory throughout the consultation, refusing to
co-operate in any display of ideal qualities. She paid
no attention to her baby, offered no apologies for her
failure to attend, and refused to make any promises for
the future. Her manner made it plain that she felt the
occasion to be a criminal trial, that she was there
against her will, and that she had no hope of justice.
As such she refused to defend herself. Nevertheless the
doctor acted with continual courtesy; and since she
failed to display 'normal' feelings towards her child or
to provide reasonable excuses for her behaviour, he
himself sought to fill the gap. Since she showed no
affection for the child he praised it in extravagant
fashion and encouraged her to do the same, likewise
offering her a long series of excuses for her failure to
attend. Only after a succession of offers and rejections,
during which it must be said he grew increasingly irritated, did the doctor abandon his attempts. Even then he
did not overtly condemn the mother, but merely said that
he would refer her to a social worker to see if she could
help.

NORMAL MOTHERS AND ABNORMAL CHILDREN

So far it may seem that any mother could be easily idealized so long as she was relatively competent, attended
regularly and had no competition from husband or social
worker. This was indeed true of a large number of cases
where discrepant information was readily avoided and
little if any repair work was necessary. But whatever the
actual qualities of a mother, certain medical conditions
posed a serious and sustained threat to the easy
achievement of the ideal. Psychiatric cases and those
of mental or physical handicap were equally dangerous, if
in different ways. Severe handicap was an immediate
challenge to a mother's capacity to cope and might also,
particularly in the long run, threaten the affection and
care that was a child's due. In psychiatric abnormality
the parents might be the actual cause of a child's
condition and, since the mother was the child's normal
manager she must, it followed, bear a large part of the
blame. Thus both types of condition created circumstances
in which a mother's character might be rewritten or indeed
might have to be rewritten if a cure was to be effected.
Here then were two serious threats to the image of natural

motherhood; how could they be met without using the
reconstitutive character-work that marked the charity
format? Since these conditions differed in their
potential effects. staff adopted different procedures
to solve this problem.

As regards psychiatric abnormality, doctors' basic
strategy within the bureaucratic format was, as elsewhere,
simple avoidance. If the possibility of maternal involvement was not mentioned, then there was no overt risk
to the mother's good name. Such a stance was eminently
plausible since these were medical and not psychiatric
clinics. There were however a large number of conditions
which staff felt to have an important psychiatric aspect,
or might on occasion be wholly psychological in origin.
Asthma, headaches, enuresis, encopresis, breath-holding
attacks; in all these cases doctors could have made
searching investigations into family life. This was not,
however, their practice, even when this aspect was raised
by parents themselves. This for instance is an enuresis
case:

    Mother: Could it be his nerves?
    Dr G: That's certainly part of it.
    Mother: Well, he was given an injection at the
            doctor's. It might be that. He's never wet
            during the day. Could it be his nerves?
    Dr G: And he's just seven?
    Mother: Seven.

The doctor continues on to other topics.

This example is from a Scottish clinic; and it demonstrates very clearly the standard Scottish practice of not
even mentioning the possible psychiatric aspect of such
conditions if it could be avoided, let alone investigating
this with the mother. In this respect there was an
important difference between American and Scottish
practice, a difference which would seem to reflect the
different status of psychiatric problems within the two
cultures. Psychiatric investigation was explicitly linked
with paediatric work in two of the specialist American
clinics, but in none of the Scottish ones. At coffee- and
meal-times some of the American staff discussed themselves, their colleagues and the hospital in psychiatric
terms. Such a vocabulary was never used by Scottish
staff. Further, while it was only a minority of American
staff who engaged in such analysis, all seemed far more
ready to talk about psychiatric matters with parents than
did their Scottish equivalents. Psychological problems
were treated as more everyday affairs, which did not

necessarily threaten a parent's good name. Thus, in contrast to the case of enuresis seen by the Scottish doctor here are an American doctor's remarks to the mother of a child with encopresis:

> Dr O: It's psychological so your paediatrician is right. There are always three things it could be. (He describes two somatic possibilities and the reasons why he thinks they do not apply here.) Thirdly, it can be a thing between the mother and the child. It starts up at around the age of two because that's when children learn to control their bowels.... Let me tell you this, we're not going to have too much trouble there. He's a normal kid. You ought to see some of the kids we have in here, so withdrawn, right in themselves. He's really fine. He's a nice, normal kid.... We've got to consider the dynamics of the situation. It's a battle between you and him. It is with all children. At the moment he's on top, but you're OK, because he's really a normal kid. It's not a conscious thing, it's unconscious, just like you can have headaches when you don't want to do something. Really, this is a pretty normal problem – well, almost.

This difference between American and Scottish staff must not be exaggerated. American doctors might mention the psychiatric aspects of a condition more openly but they did not investigate them, while they also minimized the parents' contribution to the problem. The condition lay in the child not in the mother. Although the American doctor described the problem as originating in a 'battle' between mother and child, the mother's role as combatant was not considered when he spoke to her. When he described the case to the interns, however, he argued differently: 'You'll find the parents in these sorts of cases are very constricted people.'

Thus, given the different status of psychiatric problems in the two cultures, doctors' typical strategies were much the same. Moreover, it was not always possible for Scottish doctors to avoid all psychiatric matters – some parents over-protected their children and required advice on how to cope with the ensuing problems, and on other occasions children were referred from the department of child psychiatry for neurological assessment – and in both these instances the doctors followed a similar line to that of their American colleagues. The problems were

out in the open so they had to be faced; but at the same
time the parental contribution to their origin was minimized.

   In summary, in both cultures psychiatric problems were
typically reified. In the Scottish clinics these things
were treated as purely natural in origin, requiring no
investigation of the social and thus moral sphere. Where
such avoidance was not possible then the problem was
reified in another fashion: by locating it within the
child and not in any wider familial context. The American
doctors were more likely to follow the second of these two
approaches, but in doing so they also took great care to
avoid besmirching the parents' good name.

   Although reification was the normal procedure for
handling psychiatric problems, there were a few instances
in which the mothers' responsibility for the condition was
directly addressed. This produced a major challenge to
the principle that every mother was a good mother, a
challenge that was met in a highly circuitous but in-
genious fashion.

   My analysis of this is based on three cases, all of
which were seen in the Scottish neurological clinic and
in each of which the doctor thought it quite possible that
a child was handicapped; but at the same time the child's
behaviour was so bizarre and the mother's reaction so
extreme that a psychiatric explanation was equally or
even more likely.

   In such unusual circumstances staff were obliged to
investigate the condition of both the child and the
mother. Whether or not the child was handicapped could
be ascertained by wholly conventional means, though it
might take some time, but the investigation of mothers
called for special procedures. The difficulty here was
that if the mother was involved - and such was the
eventual decision in all three cases - then it was essential to get the mother to see herself as part of the
problem, but to do this was to engage in reconstitutive
work.

   The solution to this problem was to do things slowly.
Whereas in the charity format mothers were expected to
plead guilty on the spot, such instant insight was not
demanded in the neurological clinic and parents were
allowed to confess over time. Further, no direct accu-
sation of guilt was ever made by staff, for the naming of
the offence and the discovery of the offender were left to
the mothers themselves. Doctors merely provided the means
to this end through ruling out organic conditions and by
giving the mothers an opportunity to talk. Although they
used social workers and other ancillary staff as their

principal vehicle for the achievement of insight, they too
played a part, seeing such mothers more frequently and in
greater privacy than was the case elsewhere. Such a
strategy was slow and often tortuous, in one case taking
over three years before it finally succeeded. The difference between the beginning and end of this process can be
seen in the following two quotations from one of these
cases, one from the first visit and the other from the
final consultation at which the child was discharged. In
the first quotation the mother defines the problem as
entirely within the child:

> Dr I: Well, what can you tell me about him?
> Mother: Well, basically it's his head-banging and his
>   shyness.... And he's got very violent tempers,
>   he screams and screams.... And he was very
>   slow to walk.... He's very loath to co-operate
>   with strangers. We can never leave him with
>   anyone.... And also he's not been sleeping for
>   two days and nights at a time.
> Dr I: Does he ever hurt himself in an outburst?
> Mother: Yes, he gets very miserable and very violent.
>   The very violent ones don't last too long.
>   We've tried various ways of handling them,
>   everything we could think of, but with no
>   success.

During the examination the child screams and fights very
violently.

> Mother: (rather desperately) This is what he gets
>   like.

A little later the child starts to scream and bang his
head repeatedly and heavily on the floor. Dr I flinches.

> Mother: We've tried everything, we've tried slapping
>   him, cuddling him, putting him to bed ...
>   (She cries.)
> Dr I: (soothingly) Don't worry about it. It doesn't
>   matter.

Mother picks the child up from the floor and both sit
there, streaming with tears.

> Dr I: Would you like to go and talk elsewhere because
>   of the noise? It's far too noisy in here to
>   talk.
> Mother: Yes.

They leave - but without the child.

The next excerpt is several clinic visits and a year later:

> Dr I: Brian has been without occupational therapy for the last couple of months and seems fine.
>
> Mother: Oh, yes, but I'm continuing to see Mrs Adams (social worker). I find her very understanding and helpful. Also, my doctor's (GP) been very good. He's given me a different drug and I can relax much more now. I just don't worry about things so much and I'm therefore not on their backs all the time and it's better for them.
>
> Dr I: And he's sleeping a lot better now.
>
> Mother: Oh, yes, there's no problem there now, if he wakes up I don't.
>
> Dr I: And the other thing was temper tantrums.
>
> Mother: They're much better now and if he does have one I just walk off and he comes round in his own time.

Through waiting and through giving the mother time to talk, her ideal character had been preserved, despite her admission of at least partial responsibility, and she herself had played a part in the formulation of her guilt and was therefore due praise as well as blame. As in more trivial cases such as the one where the mother had overfed her baby, her guilt was placed firmly in the past. It was the present and the future that counted, and in these she was clearly now a good mother, ideal like any other.

This emphasis upon waiting, allowing mothers to make their own judgments in their own time, was also the standard strategy in cases of severe handicap. But since such cases threatened mothers' ideal nature in a very different way, the strategy was adjusted to suit these special circumstances. In some respects the problem was reversed. In psychiatric cases, staff either avoided the question of the mother's guilt or else were forced to demonstrate it. By contrast, handicap was not a question of guilt but a challenge to a mother's capacity to cope with and love her child.

Such a challenge could not be avoided; indeed, it grew as the years went by and the gross nature of a child's abnormality was revealed. The most severely handicapped babies often looked little different from other babies, regardless of the severity of their condition, and many made no special demands upon a mother. But such a five-year-old might at one extreme be almost literally a monster: grotesque, violent and uncontrollable; or else, at the other extreme, a mere vegetable: immobile, passive and noiseless. In consequence, staff held that very severely handicapped children made demands upon parents which they could not, in the long run, be reasonably expected to meet. The 'natural' duties and feelings of a mother towards her child were predicated on the assumption that that child was normal, and those mothers of grossly abnormal children who could cope no longer did not thereby impugn their good name; indeed for a mother to persist in coping with her child alone was devotion beyond the call of duty, perhaps even foolhardiness.

   It might seem that such conditions presented no great threat to a mother's idealization. However, the exception that staff could make so easily was not a matter of everyday routine for mothers. Doctors had seen many such cases and, knowing the difficulties, were only too ready to suspend the rule. But for many mothers, as Voysey (1975) has shown, that rule had a universal application and the gradual realization that they could not cope and did not always love was the most terrible challenge to their sense of self. There was in consequence a major conflict between the viewpoint of staff and that of mothers. Staff felt obliged to inquire whether mothers were coping in order to provide help where necessary, but mothers could read this as reflecting upon their competence. At the same time, many mothers took years to accept fully the nature of their child's handicap. This made any discussion of how they were coping doubly difficult, for staff's discussion of these matters necessarily formulated either the mother or the child as possibly abnormal. In consequence, although for rather different reasons, staff adopted a similar strategy to that used in the investigation of psychiatric abnormality; they waited and they offered mothers the chance to talk, but they did not enforce such talk upon them.

   To show how once again such a strategy could effect change without confrontation, I have chosen three extracts from a case that was seen throughout the three years of the study and which posed this dilemma in an extreme form. The child was three years old at the time of the consultation quoted below and suffered from a metabolic disorder which caused gradual deterioration and eventual death. Despite her daughter's grotesque appearance and behaviour, the mother was unwilling to accept that she was abnormal. On this particular visit the child had run amok, screaming and fighting uncontrollably. Eventually she had been slapped hard by the father, a most unusual event in the clinic; and after this incident the doctor tried to raise the general problem of coping:

Dr I: She's always on the go, isn't she? Is she always
       like this? I mean, is this typical - it's not
       just this afternoon?
Father/Mother: It's typical.
Dr I: And you can cope?
Father: Yes.
Mother: You get used to it.

Since the parents failed to respond to the doctor's
offer, he turned to other issues. Next time, six months
later and in the face of similar behaviour, he raised the
matter again, using the same non-committal terms. On this
occasion he called the child 'quite a handful', and was
met by a similar refusal to discuss the topic further.
But three years on and five more visits later the picture
was very different. The parents enter and are greeted by
the doctor.

Dr J: How has she been?
Mother: Oh, much worse since she's been at home. (The
        child had been in care while the parents were
        on holiday.) We're having to feed her now
        ourselves. It's very difficult.
Dr J: And what about her sleep? Is she sleeping now?
Father: No, she didn't get any sleep last night.
Dr J: So, how's she been generally then?
Father: Well, she is much stronger now.
Dr J: Is she more difficult to handle now?
Mother: Yes, very much more difficult.... The nurses
        said it took two of them to bath her. I mean,
        how can anyone cope with her? The main problem
        that we have been having is with her feeding.
        You get very frustrated when you can't do it
        and you end by smacking her. I smacked her
        across the face the other day and it's just not
        fair to her. I can well understand why
        children do get battered. You just lose
        control. You just get so angry and I get
        frightened about what I'm going to do to her.
Dr J: Yes, I can understand, I understand how you can
       feel like that.

This last passage contains several noteworthy features.
In such cases doctors typically began the consultation, as
here, with an open-ended question as to how the child had
been getting on. This allowed mothers, if they so chose,
to discuss any problem that had arisen and gave them the
chance to control at least part of the agenda. And yet
in the case of this child as in many others it took some

years before the mother responded to the invitation.
Doctors let mothers decide when their normal duties were
no longer appropriate. That such a decision had finally
been taken is evident here, for the parents' ability to
cope was not just a side-issue, one raised gently by the
doctor and dropped by the parents, but had become almost
the only issue, one that the parents raised at the
beginning of the consultation and which dominated it
throughout. Note also the mother's emphasis that this
was not just a question of their own capacities but of
the ability of any adult to cope. Since all could now
agree that the child was abnormal her own status as a
normal mother was no longer in question. She could thus
freely confess to the most violent feelings and actions,
for here that confession could be followed immediately by
medical absolution. With such an unnatural child the
mother's reactions were now only natural.

Thus, simply by waiting, doctors were able to preserve
the ideal image of motherhood that was required by the
bureaucratic format. The grave threats posed by psychiatric abnormality and mental or physical handicap could
be met by letting mothers do the reconstitutive work, at
their own pace and in their own words.

THE LOVING BUT INCOMPETENT FATHER

So far I have talked solely about mothers; but other
sorts of adult might occasionally represent a child, or
at least be present in the consultation, and these too
need a mention.

Fathers provide an especially interesting case for
examination, despite the relative infrequency of their
attendance - for they themselves brought a child to a
clinic on only 18 occasions, (5) though they did accompany
their wives at a further 107 consultations.

A consideration of the role ascribed to fathers throws
some light on a common version of fatherhood in our
culture, but may also help us to comprehend that image of
the ideal mother that was so central to the bureaucratic
format, for the deficiencies that were found in fathers
reveal what was merely assumed about mothers. The very
naturalness of the qualities with which mothers were
overtly endowed meant that there was no need for their
discussion. For example, although the children's clinics
run by the Scottish and American city authorities both
engaged in routine developmental assessment, in no
instance were mothers praised for the health and cleanliness of their babies, or for their devotion, or for the

speed with which their children had progressed. Just as
failure was glossed over, so too was success. In the
natural order of things every mother naturally succeeded
and their competence and motivation were neither criticized nor commended, but simply assumed.

No such overt assumptions were made about fathers.
Their character as human beings was not questioned but
their qualities as regards children were strictly limited
- or so they were treated. While their capacity for love
was not openly doubted, a display of affection was an
occasion for some comment: 'She's daddy's girl', or 'He's
daddy's boy'. Such remarks were never made about mothers;
that every child was mother's child went without saying.
Even if father was unusually loving, he was normally
treated as incompetent and irrelevant. When mothers
attended clinics by themselves almost no reference was
made to their husband's existence. Staff did routinely
ask about the father's health, age and employment, but
the information required was typically minimal and for
the record only. Beyond this they made little inquiry.
Nor were mothers normally asked what father thought about
things or about his relationship to the child, the only
exception being cases of handicap; but even here staff
were only interested if the father's attitude was of
concern to the mother, his own feelings were not normally
treated as of importance in themselves. Similarly, just
as staff made little reference to fathers, so did the
mothers themselves. Not only did staff treat mothers as
entirely competent to answer their questions, but mothers
typically answered in the same fashion. The following
instance was the only occasion on which a mother indicated
that her husband and not herself was competent in these
matters:

Dr H: How many (tablets) does he get?
Mother: Ah! That's my husband's department.

When a couple did attend a clinic together, staff
placed fathers in a subordinate position to their spouses.
Questions were asked directly to the mothers and, though
fathers sometimes added their own comments to which staff
might reply, they normally returned to the mother for
their next question. Most fathers accepted their fate
readily enough; indeed, one even asked permission to be
present: 'Is it all right if I watch?' Watching was in
fact what most fathers did, along with minding the
children while their wives talked to the doctor. In only
one instance did a father claim priority for himself,
though some, as we have seen, quarrelled with particular

statements made by their wives and a few regularly
demanded a more equal treatment of their own opinions.
The infrequency of such assertion was at least partly due
to the subordinate position in which fathers were placed.
Staff might not openly intervene to back one side or
another when parents disagreed. But, since their attention was directed primarily to the mothers, those
fathers who had a lot to say had usually to interrupt a
running conversation. The structure of the situation
automatically defined them as rude and inconsiderate: a
fact which such fathers usually acknowledged with grins
and apologies. Moreover, their claims to competence could
be readily undercut by mothers, given a medical audience
who tacitly validated the mothers' authority. (6)

Having considered the general absence of fathers from
clinics and their subordination to their wives when they
did attend, one may now turn to those rare occasions when
they were a child's sole representative. Since on these
occasions at least they could not be excluded from the
conversation, such meetings are unusually revealing about
the identity which staff ascribed to fathers. First,
given the rarity of the event, it typically produced some
comment and speculation, as the following quotation illustrates:

Dr G: Now this (file) is the new patient.
Nurse: It's the father who's come up with him today.
Dr G: Uh-huh. I wonder why it's always the father.
His father brought him to the GP, so the GP
noted. The father brought him here today ...
(pause) ... Father is taking on the maternal
role today then. Or rather, I suppose it's all
part of the merging of roles that's going on
these days ... (pause) ... Mind, they're still
not very good at giving histories.

After the consultation:

Dr G: That young man wasn't too bad. He was a bit
vague and a bit glib. He was overdramatizing the
situation and he was obviously trying to please
me. He said 'Yes' when he wasn't quite sure....
Fathers often want to please you. They tell you
what you want to hear. They don't realize the
importance of it. They think it's like a chap in
the family asking questions about finance; any
answer will do.

Fathers then had distinct drawbacks when called upon to

act as a child's medical representative. But many mothers were also held to be inadequate and, as has been seen, this did not prevent their idealization. With fathers it was different. Whereas mothers' competence was never openly questioned, this was almost a matter of routine for fathers. Ten out of the thirteen fathers were clearly treated as both substitutes for their wives and rather poor ones at that. ⌐The incompetence ascribed to them did not, however, affect their good character. They might not be the ideal representative for a child, but it was also made explicit that this was not a duty to be expected of a father. Staff did not question their character, merely their knowledge of the child.

To begin with, staff routinely inquired about the father's wife. Mothers were not expected to account for the absence of their husbands but fathers were often asked this, either directly, or rather more tactfully the question might be put to the child instead: 'Has mummy come today?' Moreover not only could a consultation not start without such a question, but it could not normally end without a further emphasis on the fact that here was a substitute. Fathers were asked if their wives had any questions that they wanted answering, or else given a message to carry home with them: 'Well, if you could tell your wife that although it may not clear up, not all cases do, but there is a very good chance.'

Apart from such indications of their secondary status, fathers were normally told that staff did not expect too much from them; and when a father did well he might be elaborately praised, whereas mothers never were:

Dr I: What was the weight at birth?
Father: 7½ pounds.
Dr I: Gosh, you've got a good memory! I expect mothers
       but not fathers to remember. It's 7½ pounds, *you
       think* (my emphasis).

One father displayed great technical knowledge about his child's condition and was able to describe his medical history in a most sophisticated fashion; but even he was treated as naturally ignorant when it came to discussing the child's present state:

Dr I: I just want to ask you a few questions about what
       Ian is doing now. I don't know how you'd manage
       since I'd have great difficulty in answering them
       myself, but let's see how you get along.

Male doctors, it seemed, might lack such knowledge of

their own children, and they did not normally expect it
of other men.

There were three fathers whose competence went unquestioned; of these, two were solely responsible for the
care of their child, the only two fathers in this position. Only here it would seem were they treated not as
substitutes but as representatives, and granted the wholly
ideal character that was given with such ease to any
mother.

GRANDMOTHERS

Grandmothers might represent a child on occasion, and in
many ways they received similar treatment to fathers.
They too only performed this task infrequently, though
slightly more often than fathers, 18 grandmothers being
seen in a total of 30 sessions and with nine different
staff members, two of them American. Similarly, they
might also accompany mothers to the clinic, though far
less frequently than fathers, a total of only six such
occasions being noted. In this latter situation they too
were accorded a subordinate role, while when they were a
child's sole representative they were once again treated
as a substitute. Queries were commonly made about the
mother's absence, and they were often asked if the mother
had any special questions or worries. Just as great affection between father and child was worthy of some
comment, so too the love of a grandmother was not that of
a mother. Where grandmothers were themselves taking care
of a child, their affection and commitment were not simply
assumed but were praised or asserted, since such responsibility was beyond the natural order of things.

There were, however, two important ways in which the
character of grandmother was rather different from that
of a father. Typically their competence was not at issue;
and their very claim to this, when coupled with their
greater independence, meant that their subordination to
the mother could not be so readily assumed. Once again
these features were displayed most clearly on those occasions when they alone accompanied the child. As mothers
themselves, grandmothers were assumed to know how to look
after young children and, as interested parties, they were
taken to know a great deal about any child whom they accompanied. Here the staff discuss the normal qualities
of grandmothers. Their talk is prompted by the total
silence that has greeted the doctor's announcement that
the grandchild is likely to be retarded:

> Dr J: I don't think they (mother and grandmother) took
>   much of that in.
> Nurse: No, and the grandmother seemed worse than the
>   mother, which is unusual.
> Dr J: Yes, they've seen more of life if nothing else
>   and they've got more experience of children so
>   they talk more.

In these ways a grandmother might make a better representative than a father. There were, however, problems,
for their ability to supply detailed, current information
might be as bad as any man's: 'It's a pity the mother's
not with her; she (grandmother) won't know much about the
case.' Nevertheless, grandmothers were still idealized in
a fashion quite unlike that of fathers. Overtly their
competence was unquestioned and this gave them the opportunity, if they so wished, to criticize the competence
of the mother herself. Only one father attacked his
wife's capacity to look after their child, and then only
on the known medical grounds of her insanity. Several
grandmothers however made criticisms of their daughters
or daughters-in-law.

> Grandmother: Well, I think he's too fat; is he?
> Dr A: Well, he certainly seems to be putting on weight
>   pretty quickly. (She then questions her about
>   the baby's feeding and adds....) Well, I should
>   definitely cut down on what you're feeding him,
>   otherwise he'll be very overweight later on and
>   his weight'll be just too much for him to carry
>   about, and it'll be bad for his chest.
> Grandmother: Aye, it must be bad for his chest. He
>   gets porridge too. His mother's not very
>   good with him. She never perseveres with
>   the bairn.
> Dr A: Well, I should try cutting the Farex out.
> Grandmother: She gave him custard yesterday.
> Dr A: That's no good either. Strained soup is better.
> Grandmother: Yes, I agree.
> Dr A: And I should cut out all the cereal.
> Grandmother: He's quite content with that.

Such comments show that when a mother was not present
her character, far from being assumed, might be a central
topic of discussion. This was particularly true when a
child was no longer living with its natural parents.
Instead of competence, care and affection being placed
firmly in the natural order of things, at least for
mothers, these were now the subject of detailed investi-

gation by staff and possible denunciation by the child's present guardians. Here for instance is a quotation from an American grandmother who had permanent care of a child:

> Dr R: What about her parents?
> Grandmother: Her father doesn't love her at all. He doesn't hold her like a normal child. He just refers to her as 'the child'.
> Dr R: Do the parents live together?
> Grandmother: Yes, but neither of them is normal.... She was very odd when she was young and then she ran off and married the father and he's just the same. They're both very odd. All his family are mental in some way.

These last two quotations illustrate a more general rule than any that have so far been considered. As one can now see it was not that mothers were always treated as ideal within the bureaucratic format; such qualities were guaranteed them only so long as they were physically present in the consultation. Rather, whoever was with the child was to be treated as of good character, almost regardless of what they did or said. The grandmother who criticized her daughter's feeding of the child had an oily, ingratiating manner which the doctor disliked intensely. She was also known by the health visitors to have neglected her own children when they were small. Nevertheless, such facts were only mentioned after the consultation. Within it she was still idealized, just as her daughter would have been had she appeared instead. This idealization differed somewhat according to the type of representative, whether they were mother, father or grandmother, but in no case was their fundamental integrity overtly doubted.

THE EXCEPTIONS

Two limiting cases to my argument should be noted. These concern, first, a child's bureaucratic eligibility and, second, some further properties of adequate representatives.

To arrive at a clinic, patients had first to come through the correct organizational channels, and all of the settings had some form of prior screening in which ancillary staff checked identities, purposes and appointment cards and, in the American settings, investigated finances as well. The patients and parents observed

in this study were therefore pre-selected, and the idealization that took place within the consulting room was
carried out on those whose bureaucratic fitness had
already been certified.

That certification was a necessary condition for idealization can be seen by examining those instances when
things went wrong, for not all the patients who reached
the doctor met the proper criteria. Some latitude was
permitted. Some mothers turned up at the wrong time or
in the wrong week but, although they often had to wait a
while, all were seen and treated in the normal fashion.
There were, however, two cases, both in the Scottish
children's hospital, which deviated far more grossly from
the standard criteria, and in these no such accommodation
was made. In one instance a casualty officer interrupted
a clinic as he could not find a doctor to warrant an
emergency admission to the hospital. In the other the
parents were American and did not realize that Scottish
hospital doctors could be seen only through referral from
a general practitioner. In both cases there was a child
with a medical problem and parents to act as representatives. The standard conditions for a consultation and
for the consequent idealization of the parents were thus
met. In neither case did a consultation occur, despite
the parents' attempts to initiate this. ʼ The first doctor
talked solely to the casualty officer, ignoring the
mother's remarks about her child; she was treated
throughout as if she were not physically present. The
American parents were talked to, but curtly and about the
Scottish medical system, not about their child. To be
treated in a proper fashion one had first to come through
the proper channels.

The other exception concerned cases where there were
serious doubts as to the adequacy of the child's representative. It has already been seen that this adequacy
was not a matter of actual character or competence.
Whatever the qualities of a mother, the bureaucratic
format clothed her in only the seemliest of garments.
Fathers and grandmothers too, though plainly substitutes,
were nevertheless idealized. But there were limits. The
first of these involved the command of English. Those who
could not speak it could not be representatives, however
admirable their other qualities. Five such cases were
seen, all of which ended in chaos and the open expression
of frustration by medical staff. The second limit was a
less technical matter. Familial substitution for a
child's mother could not go beyond fathers or
grandmothers, any further was illegitimate and a parental
dereliction of duty. In such circumstances the unfortu-

nate substitutes, far from being idealized, could be
openly criticized, along with the parents who had sent
them.   Only two such cases were observed, but they were
also the only two occasions on which familial substitution
went beyond the normal bounds.   In one American hospital
clinic the mother had sent a neighbour; while in a
Scottish hospital clinic an elder brother aged around 20
made do for the child's parents.   Both were treated in a
fashion quite unlike that accorded to other representatives within the bureaucratic format.   The brother says
his parents cannot come because it would mean bringing
their baby girl out in cold weather.

> Dr J: Well, I don't think I'll be able to get anything
>   in the way of a good history without them.   (This
>   is a referral for suspected epilepsy.)   I'll try
>   something.

The doctor asks the child about the fits, but she can
remember nothing.   The doctor repeats that it is difficult
to get a good history under these conditions.

> Brother: (truculently) But you can't bring a baby out
>   in this kind of weather.
> Dr J: Oh, well, I suppose we'll just have to soldier on
>   and do our best.... What was her weight when she
>   was born?
> Brother: I don't know.
> Dr J: And when did she sit up?
> Brother: At the normal stage, I think.
> Dr J: Well, if you don't know there's no point in
>   guessing. When did she walk?
> Brother: (truculently) I don't know.
> Dr J: Oh, well, I think we'll just have to give this
>   up.

In fact this consultation trickled on for some time,
though with little more progress being made and with no
increase in cordiality.
   Limiting cases such as these were exceptional, but they
have great analytical value.   They show clearly that the
ideal character normally ascribed to a child's representative was not simply a matter of staff's personality.   It
was not the case that some doctors were naturally courteous and automatically idealized every adult who accompanied a child.   The vast majority were so transformed, but
only in so far as they met certain specifiable criteria.
Those who did not were treated in a different fashion.
They were not condemned as in the charity format, but

they might well be ignored or their inadequacies spelt out
and the consultation abandoned or postponed. Idealization
was the general rule, but it was not for everybody; and
where participants could not be properly idealized the
whole encounter was in jeopardy.

4 Collegial authority

Mothers, and most of the other adults who might normally represent a child, would seem to have done well out of the bureaucratic format. But so far my description has only been partial, for within the format each participant had several contrasting identities. Mothers were not only mothers; they were also subordinates. In regard to their children they were authorities of unblemished character and competence, but as regards medicine and their relationship with staff, they were granted no such authority. Their idealization as naturally loving and able was thus counterposed by an equivalent idealization of their medical ignorance. However much medical knowledge mothers had, or thought they had, they were almost universally treated as technically incompetent. Correspondingly, whatever the actual knowledge or competence of staff, in practice they both assumed and were granted the mantle of expert.

These twin identities form the subject of this chapter. In it I examine, in so far as they can be separated, the procedures through which staff's expertise was idealized and the methods which dramatized the ignorant and subordinate status of the child's representative. The chapter ends with an analysis of those situations which presented the greatest threat to staff's authority, and of the ways in which these challenges were overcome.

EVERY DOCTOR A GOOD DOCTOR

The idealization of staff's technical competence within the bureaucratic format had two distinctive features. First, this character was given quite unequivocally; expertise was displayed rather than proved. In the Scottish clinics, doctors' status was warranted simply by their being there, dressed in white coats or dark suits, seated behind desks and being spoken to in a deferential manner by other staff. Second, this expertise had a 'collegial' rather than an individual character. Doctors were expert because they belonged to an expert profession. In this version, hospitals and clinics were staffed by a uniform body of professionals, each one competent and all with equal access to a standard body of medical knowledge.

The principal method by which individual staff came to represent this collective wisdom was that of avoidance. Just as mother's character and competence went uninvestigated and was thus simply assumed to be good, so the staff's actual competence was ignored. Typically no mention was made of their names, mandate, training or special interests. No patient ever asked a member of staff where they had trained, what were their precise qualifications, where they had worked before, how many publications they had got, or how long their studies had taken them. More particularly, no parent ever asked how much experience the doctor had in cases of this type. The unimportance of the doctors' biography was summed up in the manner in which introductions and greetings were typically done. Although doctors greeted mothers by name as they arrived, they rarely named themselves. Naming the mother was more than polite, for it had an important organizational purpose. In doing this, doctors could check that this was indeed the person they thought it was. Naming themselves had no such bureaucratic relevance.

This impersonality extended beyond name and personal history to cover the clinic's remit, the doctor's own powers within it, and the history of the service. For example, because they had no power to prescribe, Scottish local authority doctors referred some mothers to their general practitioner, but they did not normally mention why they did so. Nor did they inform parents as to the origin or purpose of total population screening, the nature of the various sources of data from which they derived their information on parents - such as the 'At Risk' and 'Handicapped' registers which they kept - or the way in which their work was supervised by a superior. Again, just as they did not talk about their own work, so staff did not compare it with that of others. The head of the Scottish physiotherapy department was proud of her policy of 'mat' as opposed to 'plinth' work, but the pros and cons of this issue were never mentioned to parents, nor were any other of the special features of the department. Such reticence was uniform in all the clinics observed. Typically, staff mentioned their particular

competence or remit only when parents asked for services
that a clinic could not provide, or else when they
referred a child to another clinic, and even in these
cases they said but little.

This idealization of the character and competence of
the staff who ran these clinics was complemented by a
similar treatment of those who saw children in other
contexts. The assumption of collegial rather than individual expertise required a general rather than a personal
anonymity. What parents thought of their general practitioner, of other hospital specialists, of local authority doctors and social workers was almost never mentioned;
and this silence was maintained even under the most trying
of circumstances. 'Not in front of the patients' was the
rule - even where there were major professional demarcation disputes, or where it was staff's job to check on
others' work. The only partial exception was the
treatment of health visitors. In three instances,
Scottish hospital doctors either initiated or concurred
in criticism of these relatively low-status staff. By
contrast, when hospital staff referred to other kinds of
staff, their comments, though uninformative, were often
flattering: 'You'll have to see Mr McIntosh (orthopaedic
surgeon) about this; he's the expert in these matters.'
'I think you should see Mrs Armstrong (physiotherapist)
about this; she's very good with children like this.'

The general avoidance of comment about other professionals is best illustrated by taking one example in
detail: the way in which general practitioners were
referred to by both staff and parents in hospital clinics.
Not all American parents had such a doctor, but Scottish
parents certainly did. It was from him that the hospital
doctor most commonly received an initial referral, and
most parents saw their general practitioner more often
and knew him better than they did the hospital or local
authority clinic doctor. Moreover, hospital doctors were
obliged to write to the general practitioner after each
visit, describing what they had done and advising on
further treatment if any. General practitioners were
therefore involved in almost every case observed in the
study, and yet they were almost never a topic of conversation between staff and parents. This was particularly
striking given the fact that clinic doctors sometimes
disagreed with the diagnosis suggested by the GP, and on
some occasions felt the practitioner to be incompetent.
Moreover, whereas clinic staff knew, if only by repu-
tation, most of the staff within their own organization,
few general practitioners were known to them. They had
therefore little to go on besides the referral note itself

and this was sometimes both brief and opaque. Was this, for example, a rebellious or prestigious parent rather than a mysterious complaint? 'This is interesting. The GP's written a letter on his own notepaper rather than using the standard referral letter. I don't know why he's done this.'

Despite such doubts, doctors normally made no inquiry into parents' transactions with their general practitioner. They asked neither what he nor the parents had said and they certainly did not inquire into parents' feelings about the relationship. There were only four occasions in which this rule was broken, and then only in part. Each of these involved a major discrepancy between the diagnosis given in the referral letter and that made by the doctor in the clinic; and in each the hospital doctor's version was less serious than that proffered by the general practitioner. Although the three hospital doctors involved did, in these instances, make some inquiry into the previous consultation, they did so in an extremely delicate fashion. They did not point out the discrepancy between their own version and that of the GP, far less did they censure his judgment.

To give an example: in the following instance the general practitioner had suggested a diagnosis of cystic fibrosis, whereas the clinic doctor thought that the problem was a worm. Given the seriousness of the initial diagnosis, the doctor questioned the mother very closely about her consultation with the GP, yet made no overt criticism. In answer to the doctor's first question the mother had revealed the presence of a worm in the child's stool, something that was not mentioned in the referral letter; but the following comments are the only references the doctor made to the GP:

> Dr G: Did you tell your doctor about it (the worm)?
> Mother: Oh, aye.
> Dr G: Uh-huh.... (He asks a series of developmental questions, then returns to the worm.) Your doctor here, you see, says that this has been going on for nine months but you don't think it has.
> Mother: Well, I can't really remember.
> Dr G: No.

The doctor asks further questions about the child's bowel and chest problems and then returns to the worm.

> Dr G: When you saw the worm were you surprised by it?
> Mother: Oh, I just felt sick.

> Dr G: Yes.   Did you think it was a worm right away?
>
> Mother: No, I thought it was slime, but when I saw it wriggling, ugh!
>
> Dr G: And did you actually go to your doctor about it then?
>
> Mother: Well, we were on holiday at the time. We came back on the Monday, I saw the doctor then....
>
> Dr G: What did your doctor say about it?
>
> Mother: Well, he said it was just an earthworm, but I didn't think it was.
>
> Dr G: No, no. All right ... (pause) ... I would think it possible that it's been a worm that's been upsetting him.

Thus, even where some discussion of the general practitioner's actions was necessary it was handled with the greatest delicacy. Even if one finds the lack of staff's reference to general practitioners surprising, it should be noted that it was only a little more frequent among parents. Whatever had passed between them typically went unmentioned. When a clinic doctor gave a diagnosis, some parents commented that this is what their general practitioner had said. More rarely, parents might cite their general practitioner as agreeing with them in order to bolster their own version of events, while three parents criticized the diagnosis that he had suggested. All these cases were again played with great caution by staff. In the following instance a child had been experiencing great pain passing stool and the general practitioner had prescribed a laxative, but on examination the hospital doctor had found a small anal fissure:

> Mother: (angrily) The doctor didn't see it!
>
> Dr J: (mildly) Well, it may not have been there then.

In line with this silence over their own and others' competence, staff maintained a similar reticence over what may be termed the 'organizational history' or 'career' of any particular case. Even the healthiest child was examined a good many times in the Scottish city, while those who had illnesses of any consequence were often seen by many different staff, all of whom might play some part in the analysis and treatment of a child's condition. If a child was an inpatient all this was invisible to the parents: just who was involved, who had noticed this and when, was not mentioned. The diagnosis was presented to parents as an accomplished fact. The processes of observation and debate which led up to it were not revealed, nor were the errors that might also have played a part.

One of the most noticeable features of the ward-round on the intensive care unit was the number of mistakes, most of them extremely minor, that were confessed as the round proceeded. It seemed quite routine to make mistakes and there was normally no criticism of those who owned up. Errors were expected, and discussion concentrated on procedures to minimize these in the future. But in clinics errors were never mentioned, unless they were grossly obvious. It was not that staff presented themselves or others as infallible but that such matters were almost never mentioned. Avoidance was the fundamental strategy used by staff to transform their particular capacities and acts into the ideal form suitable for consultations within the bureaucratic format.

That such a strategy was accepted by parents is well brought out in the following two instances, which illustrate just how far the anonymity of such medicine was treated as purely natural. The first quotation comes from the end of a consultation which has lasted half an hour. Only then does the mother reveal that she does not know just who she is talking to:

> Dr I: What was Dr Maxwell (child psychiatry) planning
>   for her?
> Mother: Well, she said that someone would be seeing
>   her. Someone interested in specific speech
>   delay. Is that you?
> Dr I: Well, I'm interested in it, but I don't think it
>   could be me.
> Mother: And the other person we'd be seeing is a paedi-
>   atrician with an interest in co-ordination.
> Dr I: That's me. The other one may be a psychologist.

This quotation has an added interest in that it was the only occasion in which a doctor discussed his particular medical interests; and, as can be seen, it was only due to parental questioning and fore-knowledge. In all other cases such matters went unmentioned. Indeed it would appear that some parents, at least overtly, did not only *not* need to know just who the doctor was but they did not even require to know *why* they were there. In the following case and two other instances like this mothers only asked why they had been asked to attend at the very end of a consultation, having already answered all the doctors' questions. It was just assumed that organizational purposes were good ones and one co-operated willy-nilly:

> Dr G: Well, that's fine. I'll tell your doctor that
>   he's all right. Everything seems to be fine.

Mother: Well, I don't know what it was all about.
Dr G: Well, it's just that jaundice can affect things
      later. But I'll write to your GP about it...
      Goodbye.
Mother: Bye... (leaves).

In this particular case the hospital where the baby was
born had arranged for another hospital, one near the
mother's new home, to follow the child up, but the mother
herself (or so it seemed) had not been informed of this
arrangement. It was nevertheless accepted with apparent
equanimity. The experts might be anonymous but they knew
best.

EXPERTISE IN THE PRIVATE FORMAT

Since the principal method of establishing collegial
expertise was to avoid inquiry into, or even mention of,
the particular competence of any one member of staff, it
is difficult to cite instances which adequately demonstrate the procedure. As with my analysis of mothers'
character, I shall therefore rely on a comparison with
another format in which the identity ascribed to doctors
was of a rather different nature.
    My description of the 'private' format, as I shall term
it, is, like my earlier description of the charity format,
based on only a very limited number of cases. There may
well be other ways of doing private medicine, and it seems
quite likely that styles of selling will change from time
to time. To repeat an earlier caveat, my analysis is not
intended to serve as a full description of the phenomenon
but aims merely to bring out the contrasting qualities of
the bureaucratic format. (At the very end of this monograph I shall discard such caution, but such abandonment
is to suit a rather different set of purposes.)
    Only six private cases were seen in full detail in the
American hospital. (1) All six of these cases shared
certain distinctive features, even though they stretched
across the work of three clinics and three different
doctors. These features were also to be found, at least
in part, in two cases in the Scottish neurological clinic,
both involving representatives who were relatively
unfamiliar with the medical system and had had considerable experience of private medicine. Although the
Scottish doctor did not permit a complete switch to a
private format, in each case the child's representative
made strong attempts to effect such a transition, and
these consultations therefore contained a mixture of both
formats.

In some respects the private format was similar to that
of the bureaucratic mode. However, although doctors were
idealized in both, the emphasis in the private format was
on the competence of the individual doctor and not on that
of the profession as a whole. Doctors within the bureaucratic format were anonymous, but here their skills were
personalized. This individual emphasis did not extend to
all of the features that I mentioned earlier. Private
patients did not enquire into staff's careers, their
mandate or their area of expertise, nor did staff themselves typically reveal this information. Similarly, the
competence of other medical practitioners was not a
subject for staff's investigation or criticism. To this
extent staff's competence rested on collegial not individual authority. But various other matters were given a
more personal treatment.

The individualization of medical competence within the
private format had a variety of aspects. Take first the
issue of the doctor's name. In contrast with the bureaucratic format, doctors routinely introduced themselves to
private patients. That this was a matter of some importance can be seen in the following quotation. Here a
child's grandmother, absent for long stretches in the
British colonies, or their remains, and used to a private
not a bureaucratic format, sought similar treatment in a
Scottish hospital clinic. Several battles were fought
over this during the consultation. In this instance the
grandmother wanted an introduction, but the doctor at
first refused to give one:

    Dr I: (to child) Can I just see you walk?
    Grandmother: Am I in the way, Doctor? ('Doctor' was
                  drawn out and said with a markedly rising
                  tone.)
    Dr I: No, no.
    Grandmother: Doctor? ... (pause) ... Doctor? ...
                  (pause) ... What is your name?
    Dr I: Dr Innes.
    Grandmother: Dr Innes.

Moreover, although a doctor's career and qualifications
might not be discussed in the private format, they might
well be on display. Doctors in the Scottish hospitals and
clinics worked in completely impersonal rooms bare of any
individual reference; and the same rooms were used by
many different doctors for their clinics. This was also
true of the main ambulatory clinics in the American hospital, and of the various city and state clinics. But
doctors who saw private patients in their own room in the

American hospital did so surrounded by certificates. They
did not point out the parchments, nor were they a topic
for discussion, but they formed a significant backdrop for
the consultation, in much the same way as the hospital
itself was duly warranted by a framed certificate.

This personalization of medical work extended not
merely to the doctors themselves but also to their
colleagues and contacts. When Scottish doctors cited
medical opinion they talked of 'we', not of particular
doctors; and similarly, when they referred a child to
another hospital for more specialist advice, they named
the institution and not the consultant and talked simply
of 'Great Ormond Street' or 'Newcastle'. But in the
private format doctors talked, not just of hospitals or
departments, but of specific experts. The medicine that
parents received was directly linked to the 'best' available opinion. On this model the medical profession was not
simply a collection of unknown experts but was staffed by
named individuals bound by personal links. Here for
instance an American doctor discusses a child's small size
with his father, a man of considerable wealth:

> Father: So it's a little too early to do this now?
> Dr O: Right. We talk about this problem all the time
>   at the moment, and I've had discussions at X and
>   Y hospital with the experts in the field. I've
>   spoken to A, B and C about it. We're all very
>   interested in it but it's early days yet....
>   Remember, it's not just me who's telling you
>   this, I've talked to lots of people who know
>   more about this than I do. (He names them again,
>   plus some others.) And they all agree that it's
>   too risky at the moment.

Not only did doctors refer to others in these individual terms but so too did parents. In the bureaucratic
format parents did not normally imply that they knew their
GP personally. Indeed the naming of GPs was typically
irrelevant, other than as a means to address letters
correctly. In the private format, however, naming was a
matter of some importance to parents; and with it went a
strong hint of both personal knowledge and an ability to
assess the competence of the doctor so named. Here for
example is a quotation from the grandmother in the
Scottish clinic:

> Usually we see Dr Charles about him. He's been the
> family doctor for years ever since dear old Dr York
> died. I don't know why Dr Charles sent me here. I've

got no idea at all. I really wanted a surgical boot
for him. I just wanted to go to one of the respectable
surgical boot-makers but somehow Dr Charles sent me
along here. I don't quite know why. It may just be
wasting your time.

Staff themselves did not actually criticize other
doctors, but the fact that they passed favourable
judgments on some indicated that there were others who
were less deserving of praise, a point which parents
readily echoed. Although none challenged the competence
of the doctor to whom they were then talking, most made
disparaging remarks about others:

Mother: The only trouble is that the treatment will
        cost so much. The most competent physicians
        aren't found in institutions (i.e. hospitals).
Dr T: Well, I don't know about that.
Mother: Well, we've had different ones every time we've
        been here and they've never been any good.
        They've never helped.

What was most striking about such remarks in comparison
with parents' behaviour in the bureaucratic format was the
typically bland manner in which they were made. To
question others' competence was not a threat to the proper
conduct of the consultation; indeed, it was even urged by
one doctor:

Mother: We liked him (Dr Levy) particularly because he
        was critical of schools and said, 'Don't
        believe what they say.' That's what got us
        here.
Dr Q: True. It's very important work the Learning
        Disability Group does in building up consumer
        appreciation. There's gotta be a dialogue, it's
        the only way.

That such criticisms were made and even openly appreciated is not surprising given the explicitly comparative stance on which these consultations were based. As
good consumers and in their child's best interest, parents
were openly shopping around; and such a position was
honourable not shameful, something to be revealed rather
than concealed:

Intern: How did you get here?
Mother: Well, he's been seeing a psychiatrist and he
        diagnosed minimal brain dysfunction and pre-

scribed X. But we also want to get Dr Stein's
opinion as we felt we ought not just to have a
psychiatric opinion.

Just as doctors personalized their own knowledge, so
they warranted their decisions far more systematically
than was typical in the bureaucratic format. Parts of
the following conversation are like a private tutorial
for a favoured, if somewhat dim, pupil.

Dr Q: If he's nearly three years behind then he should
be in a full-time class with special education,
but perhaps we can explain why he was doing OK
in the nursery. (Turns to researcher.) Do you
know the work of Piaget?
Researcher: Yes.
Dr Q: (to parents) Piaget is a Swiss psychologist.
He's a far brighter man than me! What Piaget
really argued was about how children started off
with very concrete thoughts and then over time
they progressed to abstract thought. What we
want to know is, why hasn't he? As I said, if
he really is three years behind then he should
be in a full-time class of special education, but
he isn't. Why isn't he? I want to know why he's
not if he really is this.
Parents: Right ... (pause ...).
Dr Q: (leaning forward to mother and speaking in a
slow, intimate voice) Now, you know what a
learning disability teacher does, don't you?
Mother: (very hesitantly) He teaches children at a
level they can understand.
Dr Q: (emphatically) That's right!

In summary, whereas doctors in the private format were
obliged to tolerate or even welcome criticism of their
colleagues and had to sell the special quality of their
services with some vigour, their expertise was simply
assumed within the bureaucratic format and was in need of
no such display. In the latter mode, each and every staff
member was almost automatically granted an anonymous but
collective wisdom.

MEDICAL EXPERTISE - PARENTAL IGNORANCE

Having considered the way in which the bureaucratic format
granted doctors a generalized wisdom in comparison with
the more individualized expertise that was sold to private

patients, we may now turn to examine parents' medical knowledge and the manner in which this was handled. As can be seen, in the private format parents assumed and were granted some measure of competence to judge the service which they received, even if they were not granted any equivalent expertise. In the bureaucratic format, by contrast, parents had a far lower status. The assumption of a collective medical wisdom and the more thorough-going exclusion of critical remarks about other services were paralleled by a systematic idealization of parental ignorance.

This distinction must not be pushed too far, for in neither format were parents themselves admitted to the medical college, and in both modes the relationship was one in which there were clear superordinate and subordinate statuses. Moreover, these statuses were constantly dramatized for, whereas staff's technical competence could be idealized through the avoidance of certain topics, the establishment of their technical authority required more positive action. Colleges may be invisible and even anonymous but they are far from being entirely abstract conceptions. In professional interaction, membership or non-membership of the relevant college is invoked at every turn. The member is required to display his authority, while the client must pay due homage to the professional's expertise and indicate his own inferior status. As Werthman (1969) has argued, every action in an authority relationship has import for the maintenance, or otherwise, of that relationship. (2)

The clearest way to demonstrate this dramatization of authority is to contrast it with the very different way in which staff's expertise was treated when they talked with colleagues. The mode which such conversations took may be termed the 'clinical format', and is well illustrated in the following excerpt, which is from a case conference in the American children's hospital and concerned an adolescent girl who had suffered severe brain damage in a fall:

Dr P: There are so many unanswered questions here. She's acting so much like children we see in here who are severely retarded; grabbing, screeching, bizarre behaviour, but psychotic too.

Therapist: I'm gonna make a very profound statement (she laughs). You've got to remember that we had a normal feeling adult and then severe damage. How much of what we see is due to her losing her spatial orientation? (She elaborates on this.)

Psychologist 1: (agrees and stresses that the child is
               having to adjust to a whole new mode
               of orientation.)
Dr P: Possibly this explains the clinging.
Psychologist 1: (describes the Helen Keller case as an
               example of this.)
Therapist: Remember that this child was normal before.
          Now she will often cling as it is the only
          contact that she can get.
Nurse: You say she's got no sight, but I think she can
       see. She must have some sight. If you put a
       ball in front of her I've seen her pick it up.
       It may just be tunnel vision or light and dark.
Therapist: We've got to find this out.
Psychologist 2: Let me disagree with Jane (therapist)
               and Roger (Psychologist 1). I think
               the sensory deprivation is minor
               compared to the brain damage. The
               reason is that the whole scheme of it
               that has been built up in her head over
               years has been rearranged. What she
               really needs is small, little steps.
Therapist: Yes.
Resident: Can I ask a question? Can I ask if there has
          been a change in the nursing staff and in the
          routines that they perform with her, because
          I think it is significant that at first she
          co-operated, but now she doesn't. Have we
          over-stimulated her?
Nurse: Yes, this could be true, especially as she's
       such a problem. Everybody is trying to help so
       we could have over-stimulated her.
Dr P: Could we look at this? The question is what is
      a nurse going to do when a child refuses food?

The clinical format was used in a variety of contexts;
and case conferences displayed the features which I wish
to analyse rather more openly than some. While the above
exchange should not be taken as typical of all interaction
within the format, it serves to highlight some important
differences between this and the bureaucratic mode.
Several points may be made. First, note the constant
orientation of the participants to a wider collectivity.
Some speakers make a direct appeal to what 'we' think, see
or need to do and all are oriented to this 'we'. Moreover, 'we' are the people here in this room, colleagues,
people of some equivalency, with an important degree of
shared knowledge and responsibility. Although a variety
of technical terms are used no one bothers to explain what

they mean; it is assumed that everyone knows, just as
they know the sort of 'children we seen in here'. The
style is essentially that of a seminar. Parents too might
strive to prove their arguments in one way or another, but
the bureaucratic format was not one in which there were
agreed standards of proof. Staff and parents, when
talking to each other, displayed no such we-orientation.
They were not colleagues but individuals, with quite
separate interests, responsibilities, competence and
knowledge, and were referred to as such.
   At the same time, although a far greater appeal was
made within the clinical format to some shared orientation, the speakers also differentiated themselves from
each other in a far blunter manner than was normal in the
bureaucratic or even the private format. All speakers
stressed their independent competence and did so as much
when they concurred as when they did not. Very few
parents stated that they 'agreed' with a doctor's
findings, for to do so implied an independent ability to
evaluate clinical data; but colleagues commonly did so.
When staff disagreed among each other they did so in a
relatively open fashion, each again asserting his or her
independent authority. The above passage, and indeed the
entire case conference, was full of remarks such as, 'You
say ... but I think', 'Remember', 'Let me disagree', and
admonitions about what 'we' should 'really' do. In consequence the discussion was highly competitive: a frequent
feature of talk between staff. Precisely because they
had some share in a common body of knowledge and a common
task, each staff member's competence was on display; and
a successful analysis of a particular case could lead to
greater general influence within their organization and
profession. Parents might seek to influence particular
decisions, but they had no such organizational interests
and they were not the doctor's competitors.
   Finally, the free-wheeling nature of the discussion
needs some comment. Dr P was in control of this meeting
and he chaired it quite firmly, but nevertheless the discussion zig-zagged from one topic to another as different
speakers brought different points to the fore. Some
parents had problems or questions that they raised with
the doctor, but in the bureaucratic format such points
were presented to him for his solution, they were not
topics for general discussion and collegial action or
comment. It was the doctor who set the agenda and controlled it with a degree of rigour that would be unac-
ceptable in most kinds of collegial discussion. As such,
parents' questions and answers were to the point, not
speculative matters intended to raise new issues, and the

conversation between doctor and parent typically had a
systematic feel, an air of logical progression, which was
absent from most conversations in the clinical format.
  This comparison of the way in which technical competence was treated in the clinical and bureaucratic formats
has highlighted the basic procedures by which collegial
authority was displayed and affirmed in the latter mode.
Additional methods were sometimes necessary to ensure the
maintenance of that authority, for the dramatization of
medical expertise and parental ignorance was to be found
even in those situations where, at first glance, one might
expect them to be absent. For example, these twin ideal-
izations were still present when doctors spelled out the
technical grounds for their decisions; indeed, even when
they denied any expertise they were still the expert.
Similarly, even when medicine had failed, or parents
thought it had, they typically made no direct challenge
to the doctor's competence, and it was often up to doctors
rather than parents to uncover such disputes as did exist.
A few parents did indeed make outright attacks upon the
doctor; but such occasions were extremely rare and the
very way in which they made their criticisms still acknowledged some kind of medical authority. Even when
parents did in fact possess some kind of medical competence, they too were normally treated as ignorant and
granted a parental rather than a collegial status. The
idealization of staff's medical competence and their
technical authority over the child's representative was
thus almost universal, though to demonstrate this and the
additional procedures that it involved requires a more
detailed consideration of the above instances; and it is
to this that the rest of the chapter is devoted.

WARRANTING MEDICAL DECISIONS

The first possible challenge to the rule of collegial
authority came from the manner in which doctors warranted
the decisions they had made; for some, but not all, staff
mentioned the evidence they had considered, its various
possible interpretations, and the criteria by which they
had finally settled on one particular judgment or course
of action. Whereas most aspects of a doctor's competence
were anonymous, here there could be a considerable display
of expertise. In particular, the senior American hospital
doctors were most ready to impart such information, unlike
some of their Scottish colleagues who produced reasons for
their decisions only when asked. These variations in
style are best shown by examining the different ways in

which roughly similar cases were treated by different
doctors.

To take one example: in chapter 3 I compared the
different approaches by Scottish and American paediatricians to psychological conditions. The quotations
cited also reveal a contrasting attitude to the use and
relevance of medical information. The Scottish doctor was
silent on other matters besides the psychological, whereas
the American doctor ranged much more broadly. Here is
another set of comparisons, this time both from the same
Scottish clinic and both concerning possible migraine. In
the first case, the doctor made only one reference to his
diagnosis and this an extremely cautious one:

> Dr G: Have you heard of the word migraine?
> Father: Aye, it's like what my wife has ... (pause) ...
>   It must be very mild if it is.
> Dr G: Yes (non-committally). It's like it, is it?
> Father: Aye.

The doctor then turns to another topic.

By contrast, in the other case the doctor produced a
constant stream of medical information and comment, for
example:

> Dr H: So there has been a family history of this
>   (migraine)?
> Mother: I used to take the bile at school.
> Dr H: And you used to take turns of bile as well.
>   Well, these are always sort of inter-connected,
>   I think.
> Mother: Is it appendicitis? I had a cousin who had
>   that.
> Dr H: An appendix doesn't behave this way. You don't
>   get a sore tummy either with appendicitis or a
>   grumbling appendix.
> Mother: It doesn't bother you chronic?
> Dr H: It was a fashionable diagnosis at one time for
>   sore tummies, but there is no real reason to
>   think it does cause such things.

As one can see, doctors who warranted their decisions
by displays of technical knowledge not only departed
somewhat from the standard rule of medical anonymity but
gave a personal flavour to their expertise that is
reminiscent of the private format, if in a more moderate
form. Such individual displays of competence, even in the
extreme forms found in the private format, did not in
themselves threaten the doctor's status as the authority

within the consultation. When parents asked for reasons
or doctors provided them, this made no direct challenge
to the doctor's superior status; for the talk between
doctors and parents on these matters was not an overt
check on staff's competence, nor an occasion for proof,
but merely a revelation of the 'obviously' competent
manner in which doctors had proceeded. That such talk
might covertly provide material for checking was, for the
purposes of the ceremonial order, irrelevant. In the
quotation cited above the body of knowledge to which Dr H
refers is clearly not one to which the mother presumes she
has access, nor is she granted any such status. The
mother merely asks about the state of the art, but only
the doctor reveals it, and does so in an authoritative
fashion quite separate from the tentative manner with
which staff introduced many of their remarks in the case
conference. Indeed, in both the bureaucratic and the
private formats doctors did the telling, parents were
merely told.

FAILURE AND THE MAINTENANCE OF MEDICAL AUTHORITY

There were, however, occasions in which parents, whatever
their lack of technical competence, might well feel they
had a right to do the telling. Two situations in particular posed a real threat to staff's authority. On the one
hand a failure to diagnose or to cure threatened the
purpose of a child's continuing attendance at a clinic.
Conversely there were some occasions where doctors felt
they could help, but where their actions were seen by
parents as potentially or actually dangerous. Of these
possible sins of omission and commission handicapping
conditions were the major instance of the former and drug
therapy and immunization were the most problematic
examples of the latter.
   Both kinds of threat were relatively frequent in the
hospital clinics, particularly within the Scottish neurological clinic. However, one of the most striking
features of these settings was how rarely parents voiced
any direct criticisms of the doctors' actions, despite the
large number of occasions on which they might have done
so. To take the example of handicap: accepting that
their child was handicapped was never an easy task for
parents, and was often made more difficult by the relative
lack of medical knowledge and capacity. A precise
etiology, diagnosis and prognosis took many years to
achieve in some cases, and often cure was impossible and
no satisfactory statement of cause forthcoming. In conse-

quence many parents disagreed strongly with the doctors'
verdict at one time or another. Nevertheless all but a
handful made no direct challenge to their authority. Most
maintained an outward pose of agreement with what they
were told, even though they might say rather different
things to ancillary staff such as therapists or social
workers. Others did indicate their discontent but typically only by non-verbal means. Such parents kept their
heads down, avoided the doctors' gaze and said little.
These indirect methods presented no great challenge to a
doctor's authority, for total assent is not always
demanded of subordinates by their superiors. The slight
distancing of the lowlier members from the due ceremony of
an encounter does not threaten their master's authority,
save in cases of explicit moral denunciation where, as we
have seen, the defendant's demeanour is all-important. In
the bureaucratic format parents could be somewhat sullen
and yet still indicate their subordination to staff.
   Medical incapacity did not therefore present a major
challenge to medical authority. Indeed, in such circumstances the greatest criticism of medical competence came
not from parents but from staff themselves. Take as
examples the following two instances from the Scottish
neurological clinic:

   Dr I: We do like to see you just once in a while. I
         think I'm a charlatan really because there's
         nothing much we can do, but we just like to keep
         an eye on things to see if there is anything we
         can do.

   Mother: Well, what's he going to be like then?
   Dr I: Well, I don't think I can look that far into the
         future with any confidence. It's very difficult
         to say. And I might be wrong because so often
         doctors can be wrong and therefore I think the
         best thing is to keep an open mind at the moment
         and wait and see how he progresses.

To say such things was to spell out the limits of what
medicine could do; but it was not to discount medical
expertise, merely to describe its potential from an expert
point of view. It was staff and not parents who typically
set bounds to medical competence for, as they were held to
be the experts, only they could know when medical
knowledge was insufficient. Such comments did not
therefore diminish their general authority. Indeed, if
one compares them with those cited in the discussion of
how staff warranted their decisions, they have a very

similar form. The parents are told but they do not themselves tell, while there is constant reference by the
doctor to the college to which he, but not the mother,
belongs. 'We' might be wrong but only 'we' can accurately judge this, or point it out.

To say this is not to claim that parents never made
any direct attacks upon a doctor's competence, but such
occasions were not only extremely rare but characterized
by major attempts on the part of both sides to limit and
defuse the challenge. As an initial example, here is a
quotation from the case of a child with sub-clinical
epilepsy. This had seriously affected his ability to
concentrate but, after a three-month course of drug
therapy, he had shown considerable improvement and the
mother now wished treatment to be discontinued – against
the doctor's advice:

> Mother: Well, I must admit I don't like the idea of
> him taking these.
> Dr I: I realize that ... but ground that is lost now
> (at school) may be permanently lost.
> Mother: Well, yes, I suppose so, but I do worry about
> it. I worry about it, if it's so necessary.
> I worry ... I mean, that he has to have it.
> I suppose he must have it, but I sometimes
> think that it is not really all that necessary,
> not really.
> Dr I: Oh, yes, I appreciate what you're saying but it
> is a severe problem when his class teacher finds
> that he can't cope, that he's not learning and
> that he's falling behind. The Educational Psy-
> chologist has checked that he has a normal IQ so
> that's not the reason he's falling behind. They
> were so worried that they asked a Child Psychia-
> trist to look into it. There's enough to be
> gained here to make it worthwhile.
> Mother: It's just a drug of course to *you*. I mean,
> you're prescribing them every day.
> Dr I: (very firmly) No.
> Mother: It's like all drugs, it's not dangerous....
> Dr I: Yes.
> Mother: If it's used properly, but we lay people do
> worry about it.
> Dr I: Yes, I know that. I'm aware of that. But it's
> not a drug of addiction. Look on it more as a
> medicine. Unfortunately we use the same word
> for both.

The first point to notice about this quotation is the
heightened emotional tension which accompanied the

mother's challenge. If one reconsiders the mood of the
case conference from which I quoted earlier, not only were
challenges a standard feature of the discussion but they
were done in a relatively easy way. By contrast, for a
parent to question a doctor's competence in the bureaucratic format was to threaten the entire social occasion.
Minor parental sniping could be done with little or no
visible emotion, but fundamental questioning of medical
wisdom, and thus medical authority, was usually accompanied by raised voices and flushed faces. It is thus not
surprising that in the above example the mother's personal
attack upon the doctor was immediately followed by a
significant withdrawal. As soon as the doctor too raised
his voice the mother retreated.

The precise way in which the retreat was managed is
also of some interest. I have noted that authority
relationships required constant dramatization for their
successful enactment. But the style in which they were
played was usually implicit. Doctors did not normally
state that they were the expert, nor did parents usually
formulate themselves as ignorant. Where there was a real
threat to the ceremonial order, then such a spelling-out
might well be done, though typically it fell to parents
rather than to staff to do this. Just as it was normally
up to doctors, not parents, to describe the limits of
their own expertise, so it was parents' task, where appropriate, to depict their own ignorance and staff's
competence. Each party then was expected to draw attention to its own defects. In the incident above, the
mother followed her direct attack upon the doctor by a
description of herself as a member of the laity. This
reference drew the sting from her challenge and enabled
the doctor to take on a calm and teacherly style in his
reply: 'Look on it more as a medicine. Unfortunately
we use the same word for both.'

This successful minimization of the offence caused by
direct parental criticism of a doctor's competence was
standard in cases of far more gravity than this, even
though this incident was itself exceptional. Even where
serious parental challenges were not overtly resolved (and
there were only four such cases in the entire study) in
three out of these four cases doctors and parents agreed
to differ. (3) The incident was treated as no more than
that: as something set apart from the rest of the consultation and in no way threatening it. Arriving at this
point could, however, take time. Here, for instance, is
a mother's denunciation of a doctor for having, as she saw
it, misinformed her of the possible side-effects of a
drug:

Mother: She took a headache on the Friday and then she
        was sick *all day* on the Saturday and *all day* on
        the Sunday and she had to stay off school....

Dr I: Well, we don't think that's the fault of the
      drug.

Mother: Well, Dr Hastings (GP) thought it was.

Dr I: Well, I don't really.

Mother: It all seemed part and parcel of it.

Dr I: Well ...

Mother: (very angrily) Look. Let *me* tell you about
        it. If I'd realized it was a stimulant ...

Dr I: Well ...

Mother: ... you were giving her, I'd have looked out
        for it ...

Dr I: Well ...

Mother: ... but you told me it was a sedative.

Dr I: Well ...

Mother: Well, I read the note in the chemist. And it
        said it *was* a stimulant.

Dr I: (with raised voice) I know, and you read that it
      was given as a stimulant to adults.

Mother: It said it was a stimulant when I read it in
        the chemist's.

Dr I: It didn't say that at all.

Mother: Well, I called in Dr Hastings and he was very
        upset.... There just couldn't have been any
        other reason for it.... There's no doubt about
        it at all.... And I'm not going through all
        that again.... Dr Hastings couldn't find any
        other reason for it.

Despite the vehemence of this attack, signified not
only by the mother's anger but by her open formulation of
herself as the one who was going to do the telling, the
doctor eventually reasserted his normal technical authority. In the passage that followed directly from the above
quotation, the doctor made an ironical but heavy appeal
to his authority and the mother immediately began to treat
him, conversationally at least, as a proper expert:

Dr I: My own feeling, Mrs Logie, for what it's worth,
      is that this illness is not related to the X.
      X doesn't produce these effects in children.

Mother: Do they not have fevers or sore throats, then?

Dr I: No.

The mother's protests continued for some time but in a
much diminished form, and eventually the doctor drew a
line under the topic and started on a fresh one; one in

which his expertise was granted its normal status: 'Well, anyhow, the present position is she's off all medicine except Y.' From then on the interaction was of a completely normal form. The mother's doubts may still have been there but they were carefully segregated. Other topics were discussed in a cheery fashion, the mother even sharing in or making a joke with the doctor on two occasions. Only at the very end of the consultation, fifteen minutes later, was the topic referred to again, and then in a way which indicated an understanding, or at least a truce: (The child's condition had in fact improved considerably since the incident and the doctor had gone on to discuss cutting down drug Y.)

> Mother: You're not thinking of trying anything else for her during the day.
> Dr I: I don't think so. Especially after this rather unfortunate incident.
> Mother: (meaningfully) Yes.
> Dr I: Also, there are one or two other things that are going to happen in the future. There's going to be her glasses.
> Mother: Yes, I think the glasses will be a big help.
> Dr I: And, you see, if she's put on the drugs today, she might start on them at the same time as she starts wearing the glasses and we couldn't really separate out the effects.
> Mother: (laughing) No.

A similar minimization, but of a slightly different kind, was practised in the only two cases where parents were openly taking their children to treatment not recommended by the doctor. These parents took pains to emphasize that it was merely a trial, that they were not ungrateful for what had been done, and that they would return if their plan did not work. Such limitation was accompanied by a similar segregation of the offending topic so that in one case the mother, after criticizing staff, gave instant indication of her continuing reliance on them. This mother was trying the Doman-Delcato or Philadelphia method of treating brain-damaged children, a non-Health Service facility:

> Mother: (aggressively) You see, nobody before Mrs Robins (Philadelphia staff) ever gave us something to work on with Ian. We came over here and you said, 'Is he getting on OK?' and that was it. My husband said when I got home, 'What did they say?' And I'd say, 'Nothing,

> just the same.' No one ever said, do this or
> do that ... (pause) ... Well, Mrs Jones
> (hospital physiotherapist) she's been a great
> help, but Mrs Robins said, 'Do X,' and 'Do Y.'
> The only snag now is getting a therapy table
> .... (abrupt change in tone) What do you do
> with all your old ones?

My final method for showing the near-universality of
the principle of medical authority, whatever the degree of
medical failure or imagined failure, is that it was staff
who very often revealed parental discontent and not the
parents themselves. Just as it was doctors who normally
set the limits to medical competence, so it was they who
quite often brought disagreements out into the open, or
tried to do so, for this presented no direct challenge to
their own authority. The following quotation concerns a
mother who had recently seen a television programme on
autism and had asked the doctor if her own, severely
retarded child was autistic. The doctor spent some time
explaining why he felt this was not the case, but the
mother made no overt signs of accepting his arguments.
Like many parents she did not express her discontent in
any direct fashion, relying solely on non-verbal means to
indicate her feelings. She kept her head down during the
doctor's discussion of autism and thus avoided his gaze.
Similarly when he had finished speaking she made no reply
at all but looked most solemn. Eventually the doctor
decided to bring the mother's discontent into the open:

Dr I: I realize that you feel this very strongly and
      that you are not convinced ...
Mother: (sharply) No.
Dr I: ... by what I say, but I am quite sure she's not.
      What are you thinking could happen if she was
      autistic?
Mother: Well, I just don't know.
Dr I: Were you thinking that if Stephanie was autistic
      that there would be a lot of things that one
      could do for her?
Mother: Well, I know that you don't know much about
        autistic children.
Dr I: No, we don't. In point of fact if Stephanie was
      autistic I think you'd have more worries than if
      she was just backward. I was just wondering if
      you were thinking that, if she was autistic, she
      was missing out on a lot of things that we could
      be doing?
Mother: Well, I wondered if there was some special kind
        of training to get her speaking?

This instance is particularly striking because outside the clinic this mother expressed the strongest criticism that any parent made during the study. A few days after attending this consultation she wrote an angry letter to the doctor, denouncing the competence of the medical staff in the hospital and withdrawing her child entirely from treatment. Some other parents stopped attending clinics but none formally withdrew in this fashion. Yet within the consultation it was the doctor who formulated her discontent and not herself; and he had to use repeated questions to reveal her challenge, stating what he thought she might think and asking her if this was indeed so.

Apart from giving a good illustration of the way in which parents concealed their strongest criticisms, this quotation also tells us something of the risks that doctors ran if they attempted to uncover what parents tried to keep hidden. (4) Although it was often doctors rather than parents who revealed major parental doubts, it should not be imagined that this was a routine procedure. Such revelation was certainly part of staff's agenda with the more problematic cases such as handicapping conditions, but it was normally practised only when the occasion seemed most auspicious – and even then the parents might not be drawn. Just as staff relied on the passing of time to let mothers raise doubts about their maternal competence, so they usually waited until the time seemed right to raise the issue of their own competence. To discuss such matters was no easy task, even if they themselves were first to name the topic. In the example quoted above the doctor's first remark was immediately followed by a display of anger from the mother; the first that she had shown in the clinic. Moreover, although she controlled her emotions after this, one of her following remarks was a more direct claim to medical knowledge than any she had made previously. Whereas before she had merely reported what had been said by others on the television programme, she now assumed a personal authority and an inside knowledge – 'I know that you don't know' – and for parents to talk in collegial terms was to threaten medical authority seriously. Although these particular challenges were successfully resolved, at least within the consultation itself, the very dangers that the formulation of discontent might produce meant that staff normally avoided it, just as they avoided detailed formulation of their own competence except where strictly necessary.

THE CHALLENGE FROM PARENTAL COMPETENCE

The final threat to staff's authority within the consultation resulted not from medical failure but from parental
competence. This was only rarely an issue. Although
mothers were granted a certain competence, this normally
related just to their care of the child. Within the
clinic, proper mothers were expected to be subordinate to
staff and few claimed any medical competence. Those
handful of mothers who did make a direct attack upon the
doctors nevertheless phrased much of their criticism in
lay terms. The mother of the child with sub-clinical
epilepsy appealed not to her own expertise but mostly to
her worries as a mother; and such worries were of course
virtues, things that any proper mother should have. In
the two other cases that I have cited the mothers certainly referred to an authority, but not their own; in one
case it was a television programme and in another it was
their general practitioner. Such references might bolster
mothers' claims, but they themselves did not speak as
members of the college whereas hospital specialists could
and did.

Not all staff could make unchallengeable claims to
superiority; and, while ordinary parental competence
posed no threat to doctors, it might be more of a problem
to staff of lower technical and social status. Doctors
never complained of being socially upstaged by parents
but, when asked what kinds of parents they disliked if
any, the Scottish physiotherapists immediately mentioned
'people who put on airs' and 'who think they're too good
for you' and, although no examples of direct parental
criticism of their competence were observed, one such case
was reported during fieldwork:

> Therapist B said that when John's mother came in she
> claimed that she could walk him better than Thera-
> pist A. So Therapist A told her to demonstrate how
> she did it and there wasn't any difference, except that
> John lurched more when walked by his mother. Ordinari-
> ly, she said, she would have been very angry at this.
> After all, what was she here for? But if it kept the
> mother happy, well, just let her go on thinking it.
> She added rather sourly that the mother kept on giving
> her advice on how to treat John and get a good per-
> formance out of him.

With doctors, in contrast, parental competence was a
threat to their status only when it was of a kind akin to
their own; and this was, of necessity, rare. Neverthe-

less, 20 cases were seen when the parents present either
had, or had access to, some kind of competent medical
knowledge. (5) In two cases the mother was a doctor and
in a further six the mother either was or had been a
nurse. Three other parents worked in medically-related
occupations and were a dentist, a radiologist and a drug
company representative respectively, while another three
parents worked in related academic disciplines. Apart
from such occupationally given knowledge, there were some
mothers who were closely related to medical experts. Four
were married to doctors and a fifth was the daughter of a
doctor. In four out of these last five cases, the relative was a hospital doctor and known to staff by repu-
tation, if not always personally. There was also one
mother who ran a local parents' group for handicapped
children and attended regional and national conferences
on the matter. Although not professionally trained, she
had a wide knowledge of many aspects of the condition
besides those which related to her own child.

Given the rather different claims to knowledge or
influence which these parents could potentially make, it
is not surprising that there were major variations in the
manner in which consultations involving them proceeded.
However, in the majority of cases there was in fact no
challenge of any kind to staff's technical authority, and
the idealization of medical expertise and parental ignorance occurred in much the same fashion as in any other
consultation. Doctors and parents stayed clearly within
the guidelines of the bureaucratic format, and the competitive, collegial atmosphere of the clinical format was
avoided.

This is not to say that these occasions were completely
identical with those where parents had no claim to inside
knowledge, but the differences were trivial. When talking
to a doctor's wife one doctor put his feet up on the table
- something that he did not normally do. In another
instance a mother who was also a doctor displayed her
child's slight cranial abnormality to the researcher with
considerable clinical enthusiasm. But in other respects
these consultations were little different from any other.
Generally doctors spoke to such parents in a slightly more
technical fashion than was usual and sometimes gave them
more time than other parents received, but their consultations normally bore no resemblance to the nature of the
clinical format. Indeed in two cases, both involving ex-
nurses who had previously worked in the Scottish
children's hospital, the mothers paid a far greater
respect to the norms of the bureaucratic format than was
found in most other consultations. What was normally

tacit was here spelt out and both behaved as if it was
wrong to ask anything of a doctor, for fear of challenging
his authority:

> Dr I: Make an appointment for me then, and I'll just
>   check her over again.
> Mother: Well, if you don't mind me asking, will this
>   take a long time?
> Dr I: Oh, well, we might have to do it until we are
>   absolutely sure.
> Mother: Well, I know I shouldn't have asked this
>   question.
> Dr I: Well, it's a fair enough question. It's just
>   that we're unable to answer it. I think ...
>   (pause) ... it might be ... (pause) ... it might
>   be a month or two.

This behaviour suggests that medical competence on the
part of parents, far from automatically modifying the
nature of the bureaucratic format, may in some cases
merely reinforce it, at least overtly. Precisely because
they were insiders and could be expected to know the rules
and their value, such parents were obliged to follow or
even exaggerate them. This argument is strengthened if
one turns to consider those parents who did actually claim
an authority in some way equivalent to that of the doctor.
There were in all six cases in which parents openly asserted a medical competence; but of these three had no
medical training of any kind but were academics who worked
in medically-related disciplines: biology, psychology and
serology. In other words, half of those few parents who
asserted claims to medical competence had no professional
training, whereas the majority of medically-qualified
parents observed the standard rules with some care. (6)
Staff's reaction to such assertion differed. In four
cases it was firmly squashed, thus upholding the rule of
their supreme technical authority, but in the other two
instances these contributions were actually welcomed. The
four parents who failed all sought to establish themselves
as independent professionals without prior invitation from
the doctor. They used a variety of means to this end: a
highly technical vocabulary; the indication of expert
action that they had themselves initiated; sceptical
comments about other issues; and offers of their own
authoritative version of events:

> Mother: I've been reading the journals and they were
>   suggesting X as a cause of the damage.... I
>   was wondering if it was something to do with

> the culture her father's been taking.... I
> mean, it's well known that such cultures can
> cause genetic change; for example, they cause
> genetic changes in snapdragons.
>
> Dr T: Oh, I didn't know this.

Despite such displays of learning none of these parents
were treated as colleagues whose professional opinion was
necessary to the consultation. Thus staff did not respond, or did so only minimally, to offers of collegial
discussion. Here for example is another excerpt from the
above case:

> Dr T: And what about your schooling?
> Mother: Well, I was at the University of X and got a
> scholarship to Y College for my Masters. Then
> I had my children and I thought, I'll do a PhD,
> but, you know how these things work out. So
> now I'm working at the State laboratory. It's
> really quite interesting work. We publish a
> lot of material. Do you know Doctors A and B?
> Dr T: No, I only know them by name. Well, well, I
> don't see any report here about urine screening.

Apart from ignoring such offers, staff also made direct
moves to define these parents as subordinates and their
knowledge as at best partial or even irrelevant to the
task at hand. One such father, as I noted earlier, was
told quite firmly that he need not worry if he was unable
to answer all the questions about the child's current
behaviour. For all his expertise, he was relegated to the
standard category of 'ignorant father'. Similarly, the
ex-nurse was told that her knowledge was only partial -
'What you're calling "petit mal" attacks' - and her professional preparations were mocked: when the notes she
had made on her child's problems fell to the floor, the
doctor commented, 'You've dropped your script.' Doctors
might use a slightly more technical vocabulary in such
cases but they took pains to indicate that their own
vocabulary was still superior. They were still speaking
down, even if they did not have quite so far to go as with
other parents.

I now turn to those two cases in which parents not only
asserted their expertise but their professional opinion
was actually sought by the doctor. Instead of having to
fight to win some recognition this was immediately granted
them, and the consultation proceeded on a basis of some
equivalence. Take, for instance, the following quotation:

Dr F: Do you think it's necessary for me to test her
hearing?
Mother: Well, I think she can hear.
Dr F: Well, I suppose I'd better just ... (does so) ...
Well, do you think that there is anything else I
ought to check?
Mother: No, I don't think there is anything really.
Dr F: There weren't any problems on discharge then?
Mother: No ... (pause) ... I was a bit worried about
her hips so I got them X-rayed, but they're OK.
Dr F: OK. So there's no need for me to do it really
then, is there?
Mother: When is she going to catch up fully?
Dr F: Oh, I think she's doing all right now. Let's
just put her on the couch. Sorry! It's just
that these occasions do tend to turn into social
chat. I don't think doctors' children *ever* get
fully examined (he grins - they both laugh).

The doctor examines the child quickly.

Dr F: She's doing fine. What's her weight?
Mother: X lbs. Why? Do you think we should be
worrying about it?
Dr F: Oh, no. It's in the normal range.

This particular mother was a doctor who was known
personally if not well by the doctor, but similarly deferential treatment was given to the mother who was actively
involved in a parents' organization. Indeed, one doctor
commented of this latter mother: 'I'm rather scared of
her, she knows a lot more than I do in some ways.'
Despite this clear recognition of both these mothers'
expertise, the form of their consultations still owed most
to the bureaucratic format and was only a partial exception to the rule of idealized expertise and ignorance.
To take the case that I have just quoted, it was the
doctor who by and large set the agenda, not the mother.
Although she provided expert opinion on various matters,
she did so only at his request. Moreover, despite his
apologies the doctor did after all examine the child. He
may have laughed when he referred to the difficulties of
such occasions but in appealing to their notorious quality
he implicitly underlined his authority within the clinic.
His earlier remarks paid due deference to the mother's own
expertise, but having done this he asserted his superior
status. She was an expert but he was, here at least,
'the' expert. Finally, the overall pattern of the consultation was strikingly similar to the general run of cases

seen in that particular setting, the special nursery follow-up clinic. The doctor's main task in this clinic was to detect those few babies who still had problems and to provide the mothers of the rest with reassurance. In pursuit of the latter aim he probed repeatedly for parental worries, although it often took time before mothers revealed their deepest fears. In having such fears and having to be coaxed to reveal them this mother proved no different from the rest.

Similarly, the two doctors who saw the mother who ran a parents' organization treated her with an equivalent mixture of deference and superordination; but again they set this inside an overall framework which they, not the mother, controlled. The extent to which these two mothers were treated as colleagues depended on the topic under discussion and, where this was the doctor's speciality, he set both the agenda and the tone of the discussion. The consultations in both these cases therefore contained a mixture of formats. Parts of them resembled a predominantly clinical format, other parts a bureaucratic mode.

Thus doctors solved the problem of handling parents who might know as much as they did by recognizing their attributes as both parent and expert not jointly but separately, now treating them as parent and now as expert. In essence, this strategy resembled the segregation of topics that was used to minimize the effects of direct parental attacks upon staff's competence. The difference was that the kind of segregation practised with the competent parent was not necessarily a matter of carefully compartmentalized blocks of interaction. The switch from one format to another could be extremely rapid, with the parents' status changing from topic to topic. Such sudden transitions demand some skill and a willingness to cooperate but, in these two instances at least, these conditions were clearly met. Moreover, even though these parents were admitted to the college, they entered only on the doctor's terms. Not all of those with likely qualifications got inside, and the two who did still paid a large measure of obedience to the doctor's authority.

5 A joint venture

So far I have concentrated on describing particular
identities within the bureaucratic format, noting how
parents received an ideal character and staff were granted
an ideal technical competence. What has been omitted is
any real sense of their joint identity, of the way in
which they were portrayed, not just as doctor and parent,
but as a team. For the patient in these consultations was
not the parents but the child, a child for whose sake both
parties were nominally present and in whose cause they
were temporarily united.

This overt alliance between doctor and parent was a
central part of the ceremonial order and needs consideration in its own right, though, as we shall see, it drew
much of its shape from the matters that have already been
considered; the form that an alliance takes necessarily
depends upon the properties of the participants.

The alliance considered here had three principal
features. First, responsibility for a child was treated,
not as the sole right or duty of the parents, but as in
part shared with staff. This joint obligation was the
foundation of the team approach. Second, just as other
aspects of the participants' character were idealized, so
too was their commitment to the individual child and thus
to the alliance. The overt aim of their actions was to
help the child, and all other considerations were secondary to this. Third, as allies who had come together in a
common cause, decisions were not imposed but discussed.
The allies might have different interests, powers, rights,
skills and duties, but progress was by agreement and not
by force. Such at least were the overt rules.

There is little to be said about the first of these
principles, the assumption of a shared responsibility for
the child patient. The mere fact of parents' presence in
the consultation constituted evidence of such sharing. By

asking staff's advice and by answering their questions, parents indicated that their child was not theirs alone, at least in this respect. This assumption was so plain that it needed no mention. Nor did it require a separate enactment for, in demonstrating their subordination to staff's technical authority, parents simultaneously granted doctors a share in the child's management.

   If the way in which responsibility was shared needs only a brief mention, far more attention must be paid to the idealization of the allies' motives. For although I have devoted considerable space to parental good character and the means by which it was produced, my account of staff's character has been partial. Whereas I have examined both the moral and technical qualities of natural parenthood, I have up till now considered only staff's medical authority and ignored the moral qualities with which they were also endowed. But for a proper alliance within the bureaucratic format both parties had to be properly moral as well as competent.

MEDICAL MOTIVES

The demonstration of proper motivation was as complex a business with staff as it was on some occasions with parents. Indeed, in some ways staff were potentially more suspect. Parents at least had 'natural' reasons for wanting to help their child, even if these were shaky at times, but the motives of staff were merely professional; put another way, it was simply a job. They could not be assumed to have a deeply personal interest in all the children whom they saw, for the children were not their children but their work; and the attitudes we feel towards our work rarely mesh in any precise way with the ideals proclaimed in public ceremonies. Concealment was therefore necessary if staff were ever to have the qualities required of a proper ally. (1)

   Let us begin by reconsidering the American case conference that was cited earlier. It will be remembered that, although there was some delicacy in what was said, the feelings to which staff were oriented were mainly professional ones. The speakers assumed a common technical interest in the case, no matter how tragic the condition and its consequences. Some were tentative in what they said, but principally so as to avoid looking foolish in front of their colleagues, or not to offend others' sense of professional pride. As the occasion was a meeting among colleagues who knew each other well, joking was in order, and was indeed a key means by which tempers were

cooled and professional jealousies abated. And, since it
was the child's condition that was the topic of conversation, it was this and matters relating to it that were
joked about. The therapist guyed her initial remarks by
saying, 'I'm going to make a very profound statement', and
laughing after she said this. Later on, when it was suggested that they get just one experienced nurse to look
after the child and that this might solve the behaviour
and feeding problems, another member of staff, an Italian
American, commented, 'What this girl needs is a good
Italian Momma - and plenty of good Italian sausage.'

Thus although the discussion was a serious occasion at
which serious matters were discussed, staff were at a
considerable emotional distance from the personal tragedy
that the case involved. The problem of how to cope with
the mother and her reactions was a technical problem.

Staff's technical interest in children may be analysed
under a number of different headings. There was, for a
variety of reasons, a major emphasis on the unusual, and
words such as 'odd', 'dramatic' or 'abnormal' were key
terms in the clinical format. Moreover, children who
could be described in these terms were 'interesting' and
might even become 'famous':

> Dr H: ... James was very well known in the newborn
> period. He really had a lot of problems. There
> was asphyxia, heart failure, hypoglycaemia, and
> he had an enlarged liver and spleen.

The initial reason for this interest is obvious enough.
Children who were normal were of no medical concern. Not
all children who were ill were particularly 'interesting',
for some had normal forms of normal illnesses. This is
not to say that a child's condition might not be serious,
or that treatment might not be difficult, but that what
was at issue was not in doubt; though here too staff were
continually on watch for the unusual or the unexpected,
even where it had, apparently, nothing to do with a
child's condition. In the following instance the doctors
had just finished discussing a routine case in the intensive care unit and were passing on to the next baby,
when a doctor commented on a note in the records:

> Dr H: That's a very funny selection of drugs for
> osteomyelitis. (The mother is being treated for
> this.)
> Dr J: (agrees and makes specific criticisms of them).
> Registrar: She's had these drugs since childhood.
> Dr J: No! That's very odd.

Staff were therefore strongly biased in their attention towards the medically problematic and those that required emergency treatment. The ward-round at the special nursery devoted almost all of its attention to these cases, while most of the other babies received barely a glance.

There were in addition several other criteria which made a child of especial interest. First, the Scottish children's hospital was also a teaching hospital, and staff were always in need of good teaching material:

Dr J: It's a beautiful example of these spots.
Dr H: They're really beautifully placed. They're marvellously discrete spots. We must photograph it.

All staff had a professional interest in the unusual cases, since their study was a central means of developing both their own knowledge and that of the discipline. Just as I myself have concentrated heavily on the unusual in my analysis of medical interaction, so staff's theoretical orientation to medical conditions produced a similar focus on the abnormal. Unusual cases might provide material for research, a key orientation of many of the Scottish hospital doctors; and they were of central interest to junior staff whose qualification as competent professionals depended on their gathering as wide a range of clinical experience as possible. From this perspective, 'problems' became 'finds' as well. In consequence, when a rare condition was discovered in an inpatient, staff might be brought from all over the hospital to view the child, and such matters formed an important topic for discussion over lunch or coffee. By contrast, children who had entirely normal illnesses might be of no technical interest whatsoever, particularly to junior doctors, as is revealed in the following quotation in which two Scottish registrars examine the files before the arrival of the consultant:

Dr 1: All three of these new cases are for bleeding, not very interesting.
Dr 2: None of this lot are very interesting. One lot of fits and the rest all aches and pains.

They start to play with the toys in the room, then abandon this and look through the records again.

Dr 2: Excitement! Excitement!
Dr 1: Yes, gripping, isn't it? (One of them selects the epilepsy case.)

Nurse: Oh, you've got an exciting one there.
Dr 2: (sarcastically) Great stuff! (Later on, however, it all turns out all right, for he returns
to tell the consultant) This boy's been having
some very interesting fits.

Apart from these personal and professional interests,
particular cases might also offer lessons in management
and provide the occasion for a review of current policy
and practice. In the ward-round at the special nursery,
staff constantly addressed a great number of general
points: when should tests be done? when should blood
be exchanged in transfusion cases? when was it worth
referring a skin condition? when should feeds be changed?
Here, for instance, the round reaches Baby Callaghan.

Dr J: Baby Callaghan seems fine. His weight is up.
He's got a rash at the moment.
Sister: I don't know how bad it is.
Dr J: There's an awful lot of thrush at the moment in
the Unit.
Dr H: (peers at the baby, then says) Have you been in
the habit elsewhere of isolating thrush? I think
I've asked you this before.
Dr J: Yes, you have. Yes, we did use to isolate it
when I was in London.
Dr L: We used to where I was in the States.
Dr H: Well, the problem is of course that isolating is
still a very controversial matter and in any case
it's very difficult here with this acute shortage
of accommodation we've got. It's been especially
difficult here, with the principle we've had that
anyone who was isolated had to stay isolated,
which meant that you used up the isolation rooms
very quickly. This needs looking at.

The enthusiasm with which doctors approached any individual case and thus the kinds of comment they made to
others about it, depended not just on the degree of professional interest it held for them, but on several other
matters also: the amount of work it would involve, its
degree of difficulty, and how this fitted into their
personal schedule. Since all patients represented work
to doctors, almost every member of staff was heard to use
a vocabulary which expressed this. Staff might speak of
'opening up the shop' or of 'getting this show on the
road' when a clinic began. If things were slack a doctor
might ask if there were any more 'customers' waiting, or
comment on how little 'trade' there was today. Where

tasks were difficult, clinics over-ran, emergencies occurred or staff were late for other appointments, considerable irritation might be displayed, irritation which
was sometimes expressed with great force. Here, for
example, is a doctor's anguished comment in the special
nursery after it had been decided to carry out exchange
transfusion: 'Oh, God! Why is it always now that it
happens! It'll mean work over the weekend!'

However, despite the heavily professional orientation
of the clinical format it would be mistaken to assume that
no reference was made within it to the more conventional
evaluations of illnesses, or that patients were invariably
treated as mere 'clinical material'. On some occasions in
the special nursery, Sister held up a favourite baby for
others to admire, and on others staff reflected on the
personal tragedy involved. Indeed, the very privacy of
a setting like this meant that staff expressed some
feelings far more strongly than they ever did to parents.
Here it was safe to criticize other services. Similarly,
doctors sighed after some parents had left, and nurses
commented on the pity of it all. Death, in particular,
seemed to provoke such language. Whereas most conditions
were simply conditions, a brain tumour was not; and the
possibility of leukaemia could become 'this terrible doubt
in the back of our minds'. Thus it cannot be said that
lay versions of illness had no place in the clinical
format. Staff took such feelings for granted in each
other; what was normally at issue were other, more professionally relevant matters. This explains why the most
dramatic language ever used to discuss a child's condition
referred to a relatively minor injury:

> Dr H: What a dreadful result!
> Dr J: You should have seen what it was like before.
> Dr H: What a mess. It's horrid, horrid!
>
> Dr J: We'll need to repeat the X-rays. That's a nasty
>   thing!
> Dr H: Very nasty.

Other babies lying in cots nearby were severely ill or
not expected to survive, whereas the baby discussed in
these two excerpts recovered rapidly. What made staff's
language so extreme in this case was that, for once, the
condition had a major personal relevance, being a medical
and not a natural product.

FOR THE SAKE OF THE CHILD

To say all this is not to accuse staff of callousness, merely to note that for them medicine was a job and thus their interest in it was necessarily different from that of parents. Although staff felt an obligation towards individual patients there were many other motives which also influenced their work: their career, academic interest, personal schedules, professional advancement, scientific development, departmental rivalry and general policy matters. All of these perspectives could be brought to bear on any one patient and each case was of more or less collegial interest as it combined these various qualities.

   Such interests were, however, not relevant within the bureaucratic format and many would have destroyed the world which it contained. Just as staff never questioned the good character of parents, so too their own motivation went unremarked. Parents were never told that their child's complaint was boring or routine, and on only a handful of occasions was any comment made on its fascination. Words like 'odd' or 'unusual' were only very rarely used, while the work which any case involved or the degree of disruption it caused were largely hidden. The existence of other patients or of other demands upon their time were not topics of conversation with parents. In all this, each case was overtly treated as a world in itself. The present consultation stood alone, detached from other medical pursuits. Staff's interest in the general was subordinated to the particular, to this child, to whom they, like the parents, were now apparently devoting all their skill and attention.

   This general strategy of avoidance fitted well enough with the medical anonymity required to sustain collegial authority. However, just as there were certain occasions when it was difficult to idealize parents' character, staff's character could also be threatened. Here too, not everything could be readily ignored, and special procedures were necessary to smooth over and nullify the more intrusive aspects of medicine.

   For example, in most of the settings parents did not see staff in private. There was normally a medical audience present, usually a nurse, very often some students, occasionally other doctors; and the simple presence of colleagues or apprentices created the continual possibility of collegial discussion between them. Indeed this was often essential, particularly since teaching was a central activity in both of the hospitals. As it was teaching that created the greatest threat to the idealized moral commitment of staff to the individual child patient, I shall treat this in detail, and this case must serve as an example of the challenge that any kind of collegial discussion presented.

Teaching was especially revealing of much that was not normally mentioned. First, from the perspective of medical training, patients and those who accompanied them were best viewed as 'living textbooks', as empirical instances of types of phenomenon (Atkinson, 1976, Edinburgh, unpublished Ph.D.). Medical problems were of interest, not because this or that patient suffered from them and wished to be cured of them, but because this was the kind of problem students were obliged to learn about. Second, medical teaching in such contexts involved the doctor's own actions quite as much as any patient's condition. It was a highly reflexive act. Not only did doctors describe the medical phenomena under investigation, they also spelt out their own involvement in the proceedings: how they had done this and why they would now do that.

Teaching could therefore be a most elaborate affair. Doctors might sketch in the general background to a clinic and discuss their general mandate, the types of patient seen there, hospital policy for these, and referral patterns to and from the setting. More specifically, doctors could detail the nature of particular problems, their various causes, incidence and prognoses, and then describe how to recognize them, the various tests to use, their reliability and the reasoning that lay behind them. Instruction might also be given on how to read a file or a referral letter, how to get a history, and how much trust to place in it. In other words, good teaching necessarily involved making explicit many of those things that were typically concealed from parents. The difficulties that the revelation of these matters might cause were presented in a particularly acute fashion in the settings observed in this study. Teaching on these cases involved hot medicine, rather than the action-replay or cold medicine found in some forms of bedside teaching (Atkinson, 1976). Here new diagnoses were actually made, fresh problems discovered and binding decisions taken.

The principal method used to overcome the dangers of collegial discussion was the careful segregation of such talk. This was done in a number of different ways. In all but the American amphitheatre clinics, one staff member was clearly in control of the interaction. In the Scottish settings, the audience never spoke to or examined the patient without the doctor's permission, and such permission was a rarity in all but the maternity hospital

ward-round. Scottish students, with this one exception,
had no right to speak to the doctor in front of parents,
save when spoken to; and the remarks made to them were
normally statements, not items of conversation which
required a reply. Medical discourse as opposed to medical
pronouncement was therefore a great rarity. The same rule
applied in most of the American settings. Interns or
residents might talk directly with parents in the presence
of their 'chief', since they had conducted the work-up,
but detailed medical discussion about the case was usually
avoided.

Such avoidance was possible because in most settings
parents and staff were readily segregated. Detailed
teaching in the Scottish clinics could be done in the gaps
between patients, while in the American ambulatory clinics
staff left the cubicles each time they wanted a private
discussion: 'We'll be back in a minute' was the refrain
which punctuated the parents' sojourn. Parents had the
right to object to teaching. One mother, who complained
afterwards to a nurse, was seen in private from then on,
the researchers too being barred. Similarly, when an
adolescent boy complained about being taught on in the
American hospital the doctor and students withdrew.

These procedures minimized the amount of collegial discussion that took place in front of parents, while some
doctors rarely ever taught openly on children. The staff
in the Scottish neurological clinic thought their cases
were too serious for overt teaching, and one of them
eventually banned students altogether. In four settings,
however - the special nursery follow-up clinic, the amphitheatre clinics, the maternity hospital ward-round and one
of the Scottish general medical clinics - large amounts of
such discussion were held in front of parents. Despite
this, staff in all these settings indicated that their
clinical discussion was subordinate to their interaction
with parents. The clinical format co-existed with the
bureaucratic format but it was a side-event. Thus, where
doctors talked with students or with other staff they
typically did so quietly and at the margin. In the amphitheatre clinic, staff discussion was usually confined to
those on the stage and was conducted in whispers. In the
general medical clinic, junior doctors who wished to
discuss their cases with the consultant waited quietly at
the side until he had noticed them; they did not themselves interrupt his conversation with patients.

Overt teaching was similarly given a secondary place.
Some teaching comments were made in ways that fitted in
naturally with the conversation with parents; the
doctors' statements serving as remarks to both the mother

and the students. Here are examples of how this could be
done, one from history-taking and the other from an
examination.

> Dr F: Is she walking yet?
> Mother: She's walking round the furniture.
> Dr F: Children usually walk round the furniture before
>   they walk properly.

> Dr F: (lifts the baby) That's a nice straight back.
>   Right! (He puts the baby back down.) Well, he
>   can sit but he's a little off balance. He's got
>   good head control. He doesn't wobble at all.
>   Hello! Hello! (The baby smiles.) You get nice
>   easy social smiles.

Such smooth welding of the two activities caused no
offence, but where staff engaged in any detailed teaching
with students something more was needed. Here they
commonly indicated that a break in the action was oc-
curring and asked for parents' forgiveness: 'Excuse me
a minute.' Such apologies were particularly elaborate in
the Scottish maternity hospital ward-round where, given
the Nightingale ward system, there was no private place
in which teaching could be done in between seeing
patients. Here, for example, are a doctor's comments from
the beginning, middle and end of a case in which the
doctor demonstrated how to conduct the examination of a
newborn baby:

> Dr K: Hello, Mrs Angus. You don't mind all this
>   congregation, do you?
> Mother: No.

> Dr K: (inspects the notes and makes comments to
>   students, then says in aside) I'm sorry this is
>   going to take a wee while.

> Dr K: OK. Thanks very much. I hope we haven't mesmer-
>   ized you.

Apart from its subordinate place being indicated, many
aspects of the clinical format were transformed when it
was used in parents' presence. As may be seen from the
examples of history taking and examination that were cited
a moment ago, staff's comments related almost entirely to
the good things that might be said about a child. Indeed,
on some occasions the very fact that teaching was done on
a child was used to indicate that there was nothing
serious at issue:

> Dr K: Don't worry. Your baby is perfectly normal. I
>   wouldn't be going into all this if it wasn't.
> Mother: (laughing) I know you wouldn't.

Even here the version of medicine that was displayed
was heavily bowdlerized. Personal challenge and enthusiasm, rivalry and career aspirations were all carefully
removed, and the resulting discussion had the gravity and
moral purpose of some lay versions of 'Science'. Such
discussion was therefore highly reassuring. At first
sight, it might seem to threaten the overt order of the
occasion by revealing what went on behind the scenes. But
the 'private' action that was thereby disclosed was of the
highest moral seriousness. Teaching might take up a large
proportion of the time spent with some mothers in the
maternity hospital ward-round but, since it necessarily
involved the spelling-out of medical practice and manners,
it could be used to display the highest motives and
principles. Thus teaching could 'reveal' that the
mothers, not the students, were the main focus of the
doctor's attention: 'It's important to get you (baby)
right up here by your mother as she's the most important
person here.' Similarly, although the baby under discussion might be used as an instance of a type, the
activity displayed was concerned with the well-being of
all. The generalizing interest of the clinical format
could therefore be shown to be relevant to a mother's
own child.

> Dr K: He's still looking a bit yellow, isn't he?
> Mother: Yes.
> Dr K: (to students) You know, don't you, that in
>   newborn babies jaundice, what we call physio-
>   logical jaundice, reaches a peak at the fifth or
>   sixth day and then goes down. Everyone says that
>   the peak is at five days but we've studied our
>   own figures and found that many peak on the sixth
>   day. So give it the fifth or sixth day. When
>   you've had sufficient experience at handling
>   these babies and you know that it's the third
>   day, if it's a mild case, you can say leave it
>   till tomorrow and test it then, but if you do
>   have any doubts, it's important to test it right
>   away.
> Dr K: (to nurse) It is jaundiced a bit. It's very
>   mild at the moment, but if it gets any yellower,
>   tell Dr James here. Otherwise we'll look at it
>   tomorrow. Bye, Mrs Morrison.

In this, Dr K not only instructed the students to be cautious, watchful and take nothing on trust, but demonstrated to the mother that this was staff's own attitude. They had not just gone along with what 'everyone says' but had conducted their own studies and produced a revised analysis. Their constant thought about such babies had resulted in better care for all. Thus, when the doctor gave the nurse instructions at the end of her lesson, her words bore a special meaning. They were not just an order but the embodiment of caring, concerned and technically sophisticated medicine. In this manner, teaching, for all its emphasis on the general, might nevertheless serve to display the personal concern for advanced knowledge that was more typical of the private format.

Although I have emphasized that teaching could be used to dramatize the serious moral purpose of medicine, it should not be supposed that all such discussions were conducted in a grave manner. Most of these clinical conversations were formal in nature, but their style could be varied to suit the occasion. Given the ineptitude of the young students who attended the maternity hospital ward-round and the normality of most babies, the doctor could turn aspects of the round into a comic turn. On such occasions, teaching was not merely subordinated to the doctor's consultations with mothers but became an amusement for mothers' benefit:

> Dr K: (to student) Now all you've got to do is to lift
> it up over here (i.e. to the measuring cot).
> Have you got the confidence to do that? Think
> how Mrs Laing would feel if you dropped him.
> Student: Oh, I wouldn't want her to be worried.
> (General laughter.)
> Dr K: (sighs exaggeratedly) OK. I'll do it then.
> (Mother laughs loudly.)
>
> Dr K: (at end) After all that the baby's fine,
> Mrs Laing.
> Student: (to baby) Goodbye (very formally. Baby
> cries.) He's got no appreciation of my skill.
> (Mother laughs loudly again.)

THE RULE OF REASON

The tacit agreement to share responsibility for a child and the joint idealization of each other's motives and skill created characters with all the qualities of allies. Appropriate identities are, however, not sufficient in

themselves to produce an alliance. To be an ally is also
to do certain things, agreement has to be reached on
specific issues, and there are various ways in which this
might be done, ways which define what sort of an alliance
this is. I have already examined one method for the production of agreement, the 'rule' of collegial authority
which clearly subordinated parents to staff's technical
expertise. This principle was undoubtedly a central
feature of the bureaucratic format, but it was not the
only relevant rule; and to understand the distinctive
nature of the format one must pay closer attention to the
way in which collegial authority was wielded.

At the beginning of the previous chapter, I argued that
not only might a variety of social identities be invoked
for any one participant in an encounter but that these
might involve somewhat discrepant characteristics. Thus,
all mothers within the bureaucratic format were 'naturally' incompetent as regards medical matters. Now, although
particular identities may have a certain independence,
when two or more are played together by the same actor,
each necessarily modifies the other. Thus the idealization of any mother as naturally caring and competent
had important consequences for the manner in which medical
authority was wielded.

This may be clearly seen by making a comparison with
the charity format. This also emphasized agreement
between staff and parents but the manner in which it was
arrived at was very different. Agreement here was simply
a matter of parental submission to a higher authority.
The oracle spoke and parents obeyed. Only the mother who
took on a 'medical student' role was allowed the privilege
of questioning and discussion. By contrast, parents in
the bureaucratic format were treated as persons who could
be persuaded, once they knew the facts. To treat parents
as obviously moral, rational and intelligent was to grant
them some independence from medical authority. Agreement
here rested on a delicate mixture of faith and reasoning.
On the one hand, parents were required to believe in
staff's ultimate authority; but on the other hand, as
sensible people who could read the evidence for themselves, once they knew what it was, they were permitted
to argue with particular decisions; so long of course as
this was done in a reasonable fashion.

The difference between the two formats may be summed up
in the terms of my earlier analysis of moral work. In
discussing the charity format, I distinguished between
face- and character-work, and noted that the latter came
in both a weak and a strong form. We also saw how the
rights to character-work varied. What was legitimate,

even a duty, for the doctor within the charity format was completely avoided by staff within the bureaucratic format. Now the right to criticize and to demand exposition is often given to only one of the participants in a relationship. One needs a social position from which to do character-work, and in many positions 'it's not your place to criticize'. In the charity format only the doctor had that place. But the bureaucratic format, by treating parents as independent, sensible and moral, defined them as clients and medicine as a service; and in service relationships the client typically has the sole rights to criticism.

In this instance these rights were not extensive. Thus, whereas the charity doctor used both ameliorative and reconstitutive character-work, the latter, if undertaken by parents within the bureaucratic format, would have undermined the principle of collegial authority. Indirect parental challenges to medical decisions were both normal and legitimate; but any suggestion of reconstitutive character-work was, as we have seen, quickly challenged by doctors and was in any case rare. Moreover, ameliorative work, though quite frequently done by parents, was carried out in a far more restrained fashion than was the case with the doctor who used the charity format. Criticism was allowed but reason ruled; and since staff were treated as entirely competent, the kinds of criticism that could be made were limited in their force.

Nevertheless, 'reasonable' parental criticism was tolerated and even welcomed, for without it how could rational agreement be reached? Indeed, parents who never had any questions and who accepted everything that staff said might be regarded as old-fashioned. Thus doctors at the Scottish hospital distinguished sharply between their urban parents and those from the remoter rural areas. Here, for instance, is a short passage from a consultation for epilepsy, followed by the conversation between doctor and students afterwards:

    Dr I: Well, I think we'll keep him on the X (drug) as
          he has had another attack.
    Mother: Oh, aye, oh aye. That's right, doctor. I
            think that's for the best. Oh, aye, he should
            be on it for a long time.

    Dr I: Well, that was a classic patient, what tradition-
          ally most patients were supposed to be like, al-
          though few are these days. That's the sort of
          patient Dr Finlay had. (2) We don't see very
          many nowadays.

Student: (imitating mother) I know the sort - 'Oh,
         aye, doctor, aye, you're right, doctor, you're
         so right, aye, you're right.'

For some doctors this attitude was a distinct fault in
their patients. Some criticized working-class parents as
far too accepting of what was said to them, even if they
did not display their agreement in such elaborate terms
as rural parents. Here, for instance, another doctor
contrasts the kind of parents found at different local
authority clinics:

Dr D: The more intelligent people tend to ask far more
      questions and they're less likely to accept one's
      answers without querying if there could be an
      alternative answer. And in this respect, I do
      think that the population who attend the Green
      Lane Clinic and some of the other ones, I think
      they have far too much confidence in us as
      doctors, they don't realize that we are human
      and we can fail in things.

Not all doctors shared this attitude. Some saw parental questioning of their decision as a waste of time,
since the parents were incapable of judging the wisdom of
any one line of action. Others expressed both points of
view, pleased that parents took a keen interest in their
child's welfare but irritated by those who tried to 'score
points off them'. Nevertheless, even the doctors who were
most dismissive of parental questioning did not challenge
parents' right to question them, merely the efficacy of
their so doing.
Such toleration was normally matched by the careful way
in which parents phrased their questions, if they had
them. As I have shown in the previous chapter, parental
questions were commonly information questions, ones which
asked for the doctor's viewpoint but treated that
viewpoint as authoritative. Even the criticisms were
normally indirect and carefully based on appeals to lay,
not professional, knowledge.
Such procedures offered at least a chance of rational
agreement being produced. Staff were sometimes obliged to
uncover criticism and certainly required to listen to it,
even if they did not accept it, just as they were obliged
to answer questions, even if the detail in which they did
so varied considerably. Likewise, although parents had
rights to question and criticize, they were obliged to
use these in a moderate form which did not challenge the
entire basis of the interaction.

This rule of reason meant that staff tolerated almost all criticism, so long as their personal authority was not questioned; and even then they made exceptions and tried to preserve some notion of an alliance. Take first the following instance, which involved a child referred to the neurological clinic for general delay, but who was still being seen at an orthopaedic clinic. The child was three years old and not walking, a state of affairs which the· doctor blamed principally upon the parents, who carried the child everywhere; blame however was apportioned only by the parents not by the doctor:

> Father: What about this leg? We come to the hospital
>   but no one says nothing about it?
> Dr J: Well, he's flat-footed but he's capable of
>   walking, the muscle tone is all right. (Examines
>   child's leg for second time.) He will walk.
>   It's just that he's flat-footed. I think what
>   we'll do is refer him to physiotherapy, umm, to
>   see if we can get him walking.
> Father: Well, I'm not complaining but I want an answer.
>   We've been coming up here for some time now.
> Dr J: Yes, he's past his third birthday, isn't he?
>   Yes, I think he needs some physiotherapy.

This example is of additional interest in that although both parents were present it was the father who did the criticism. Such a division of labour was typical of many couples. Although mothers attended far more often by themselves, there were many cases in which it was commonplace for criticism or detailed questioning of staff to be done only on those infrequent occasions when fathers also attended. If it was the father who complained about other services, or demanded to know if a child would ever walk, or what the problem really was, then such questioning, however direct, posed only a marginal threat to the central relationship, that of doctor and mother. Their alliance was still secure, for the criticism was done by an outsider, someone with no great knowledge of either the child or the clinic.

Third parties were not the only means of rendering parental criticism more acceptable. Special circumstances could also minimize the gravity of any offence. Particular latitude was given to the parents of severely handicapped children. Indeed, as we have seen, doctors actively searched for any difficulties that they were experiencing. In the following instance the doctor listened calmly and seriously to the mother's criticisms. He did not join in with all the mother had to say, neither did

he dissociate himself entirely from it. He nodded at
various points and generally gave the impression that her
problems or criticisms were either reasonable or intelli-
gible, that he quite understood why she felt like this:

> Dr G: We did talk at one time about the special school
>   at Atholltown, but nothing came of it, did it?
> Mother: It all fell through. Nothing happened.
> Dr G: No.
> Mother: They didn't want her.
> Dr G: It may have been the distance.
> Mother: It was a fantastic distance.
> Dr G: Yes.
> Mother: If only there was a school near the city, I'd
>   like that.
> Dr G: All right, then. We'll just have to see. Is
>   there anything else that you'd like to bring up?
> Mother: No. Miss Sutherland (area social worker) said
>   that she didn't know what to do with her.
>   Well, she's a dead loss. She comes every month
>   but, I mean, she doesn't know what to do with
>   her.
> Dr G: Uh-huh.

The strong concern to demonstrate agreement meant that
even major parental revolt could be rewritten after the
event. I have already noted the way in which direct parental challenges to the doctor's authority were segregated and their overall effect minimized. What was even
more striking about some revolts was the great efforts
made by both parties to translate them into an agreed plan
of action. Thus parents who sought alternative treatment
to that which they were offered were typically incorpo-
rated within a shared agenda. Take the following
instance, the only example in the study where a mother
asked for another medical opinion. Despite its rarity,
and despite the fact that the mother twice asked for a
second opinion, first from the senior neurologist in the
adult hospital and then from a London specialist, the
request was still managed with great delicacy by all
parties. The mother presented her demands as coming, not
from herself, but from her family, and observed the
greatest courtesy towards the doctor; thanking him pro-
fusely once he had agreed to a referral, apologizing for
her actions, and even offering to pay: 'Money is no
object.' This enabled the doctor to be polite in his
turn and to present the referral as a jointly agreed
decision.

Dr J: You mentioned last time that your husband was a
      bit unhappy, that he wants a second opinion.
      I've discussed this with Dr McAllister and he and
      I are quite happy for you to have a second
      opinion.... Would you like me to write to the
      London hospital?
Mother: Yes, that would be very nice if you could.
Dr J: If we feel it is going to be a help we don't
      hesitate to ask the advice of other centres. We
      can't guarantee that this would help but it will
      certainly help in the sense that it should
      satisfy you and your family.

A little later in the consultation the decision has
become a joint action, not an individual one, and one in
which, as usual in the format, the doctor has the major
say:

Dr J: Well, as I said, I think we are clutching at
      straws a bit but I think we just have to try.
Mother: I'm sorry to be such a pest.
Dr J: No, that's all right. You're asking just the
      questions that you should be asking, that any
      mother should ask.... I do think that if we get
      nothing from the London hospital we shouldn't
      bother with anywhere else.
Mother: No.
Dr J: There's nowhere else to go really.
Mother: It's very hard to take in.
Dr J: I know, it's very difficult.

A similar incorporation of revolt occurred in the
majority of these Scottish cases where the parents sought
treatment outside the National Health Service. During
the study, an American film which made large claims about
the Doman-Delcato method of treating brain-damaged
children was shown on British television, and this resulted in a large amount of publicity in newspapers,
magazines and other televised programmes. As a result,
several parents of handicapped children became interested
in the method, even though the treatment was available
only in the private sector and was viewed sceptically by
hospital staff. This major challenge to medical authority
was resolved in all but one case, with both parties con-
tributing equally to this. Far from being a threat to the
alliance, it was transformed into something which the
allies considered together. One couple did in fact with-
draw their child from the clinic without mentioning their
disagreement in the consultation, but in five other cases

cases parents raised the topic themselves and asked the
doctor's advice. In doing so, they still treated the
doctor as the authority and allowed him in turn to treat
their ideas as reasonable. Thus in the one case where the
parents openly tried the Doman-Delcato treatment it became
an experiment, something which they did with his blessing
and on whose progress they reported at regular intervals.

REACHING AGREEMENT

So far, in considering the way in which alliances were
actually made and agreements reached, I have emphasized
the special stress that the bureaucratic format placed on
the rule of reason. Clinics offered a service and clients
had rights to rational criticism and discussion. Staff
did not simply impose their views upon parents. But
reaching agreement was a rather more subtle process than
I have made out. Alliances cannot be made solely out of
debates, however reasonable their form and tone. What is
never mentioned is often as important as what is said, and
just when things are spoken is equally crucial. Such
considerations apply with all the more force to matters as
delicate as the health and future of children. Although
overt agreement was essential if the alliance was to be
maintained, it would be wrong to imagine that this was
actively sought on each and every occasion. Moreover,
although parental questioning of staff was from one perspective a search for agreement, the seeking, finding and
display of consensus was primarily a task for staff. It
was largely staff's decisions that were at issue, and it
was they who controlled the agenda and set the tone of the
occasion. In consequence when agreements were sought, it
was staff who did most of the searching, whereas so far I
have emphasized actions that were principally initiated by
parents.
    Before going on to consider the different ways in which
staff sought agreement, I must note two points. First,
the debate in clinics did not concern some abstract proposition but a particular child in whom most parents had
made a heavy emotional investment. Second, the children
were conversationally endowed with a variety of special
properties which distinguished them from adults. Ignorant
and messy, but intelligent, amusing, joyful and wonderful;
these were the essential properties of children in the
everyday usage of the clinic. As such, these were the
terms in which any discussion of a child's medical
normality had necessarily to be argued:

>   Essential normality cannot be demonstrated by a doctor
>   merely ticking off a child's accomplishments on some
>   standardized check-list, although such work is a
>   routine part of assessment, but must be directly ad-
>   dressed and established by the entire manner in which
>   the child is treated. The doctor has to demonstrate a
>   correspondence between the clinical version of normal
>   childhood and the everyday version. To treat the
>   occasion solely in a clinical fashion would not be to
>   establish the child's normality in the everyday world
>   (Davis and Strong, 1976b, pp.158-9).

This passage describes the task facing a doctor engaged
in developmental assessment, but the same principle
applied whatever the medical work or the condition of the
child. The entire manner in which the doctor discussed a
child with its parents reflected on its medical status and
was therefore a central method through which debate proceeded. Since its formulation of the child was necessarily indirect, it served as a delicate means for setting the
boundaries for more overt discussion. Where a child's
condition was held to be serious, then a relative absence
of wonderment and laughter by staff could indicate that
this was a child for whom marvelling and fun were not
wholly appropriate. Conversely, where staff held parents
to be worrying without real need, great jollity helped to
banish those doubts.

In some consultations such indirect methods were the
only ones used to reach and demonstrate agreement. In the
developmental screening carried out by the local authority
and city clinics, children were not there for the solution
of particular problems. Most mothers assumed that their
children were normal and doctors likewise held that most
were right in this belief. Given this shared assumption,
there was no need to spell out their agreement in the
matter. Indeed, to search for agreement would have been
to imply that there might well be cause for disagreement.
Staff and parents simply treated the children as 'lovable
rascals', and the jolly discussion of their rascality
served to indicate their medical normality.

Where a child came to a clinic with a specific problem,
that problem had to be directly as well as indirectly
addressed, and use was made of more formal procedures for
seeking agreement on staff's decisions. Take first the
occasions when parents were assumed to be deeply worried
about a child, but staff had few such doubts. Apart from
adopting the jolly air that suited a normal child, staff
searched actively for parental fears and knocked them
promptly on the head when they surfaced. Given their as-

sumption that the deepest worries were often the hardest
to reveal, staff often asked the same question several
times in order that every fear might be dispelled and
complete agreement reached on the child's normality.   In
the following quotation from a follow-up clinic, the
doctor asks the mother four times if she has any problems
or worries - and only at the fourth time of asking are the
mother's fears revealed. Her baby had been kept in the
special nursery at birth and was thus initially certified
as medically problematic. The doctor's task was therefore
not just to convince himself of the child's normality but
to convince the mother as well:

> Dr F: How old is your son now? Nearly one, isn't he?
> Mother: One more month.
> Dr F: Good. Have you got any worries about him?
> Mother: No.
> Dr F: So there are no problems?
> Mother: No.
> Dr F: He's eating the same food as everyone else?
> Mother: Yes.
> Dr F: Does he have any extra vitamins?
> Mother: No.
> Dr F: Has he got any other problems? I know you had
>   him in here for quite a long time with rhesus
>   problems.
> Mother: No, he's all right now. He's been OK for a
>   long time. He does have some problems with his
>   teeth - but he seems OK. He dribbles a lot.
> Dr F: Uh-huh. That'll be due to his teeth.

The doctor then asks a series of developmental questions
and the mother says the child is doing fine.

> Dr F: So there are really no problems?
> Mother: No ... (pause) ... Well ... he is small, well,
>   I think he is but no one believes me.
> Dr F: Well, he's small*ish* ... (pause) ... What's his
>   weight? (Mother gives it.) Well, he's *well*
>   within the normal range....

This 'search and destroy' method for reaching agreement
rested on the standard assumption of medical expertise and
parental ignorance. Parents produced the worries, though
often with guidance, and the doctor dispelled them. A
second method was that of conferring a joint expertise
upon parents. In this, mothers and fathers became
colleagues who clearly agreed with doctors and validated
their opinion. Such granting of medical authority did not

threaten the doctor's own status, since he alone had the
power to confer it, and it was merely a temporary
phenomenon. Where a child was considered to be healthy,
this procedure could be used with considerable rapidity
and ease. Here a doctor makes 'guesses' and then 'checks'
them with the mother:

> Dr F: And is he standing and walking?
> Mother: Yes, though not so much as she does.
> Dr F: So, despite the fact that she's smaller she's
>   ahead by about ... well, I would guess three or
>   four weeks?
> Mother: Yes.

Similarly, Dr F, in such cases, could overtly discharge
a child as much on the parents' authority as on his own:

> Dr F: Well, if you've no worries about him?
> Mother: No.
> Dr F: Then I've no worries about him. What about his
>   teething?
> Mother: Yes, he is.
> Dr F: Yes, I can see he's a handful. Well, I don't
>   think there's any need to see him again if you
>   don't think so.

In this case and the preceding instances, the doctor's
aim was to normalize the children, to indicate that they
were fine and healthy. But the procedures that were used
to reach agreement here, the search for doubts and the
appeal to joint authority, were equally suited to occasions when a child was in fact ill. In these circumstances any parental worries that were uncovered could
now serve as grounds for the doctor's own doubts. Both
staff and parents could be shown to agree that there was
something wrong. Where the diagnosis was relatively
trivial and easily treated, this appeal to a joint
authority was easy enough. Where neither of these
conditions was satisfied, reaching agreement became far
trickier. Doctors used the same methods but they did so
in much more cautious ways.
  For example, in cases of delay where parents had
already mentioned their own grave doubts about a child,
doctors often referred to these when giving their own
version: 'Well, I don't know if I've got anything to tell
you that you don't know already.' Conversely, if parents
had given no indication of any such worries then doctors
would normally ask for these. Before he gave his own
version of the child one doctor routinely said to such

parents, 'How do you yourself feel about John?' speaking
the words slowly and seriously and looking them full in
the face. Coming after the history and the examination,
such a manner indicated that the occasion was a serious
one and that now was the time to reveal any deep anxieties
about a child. Other doctors asked parents for such
comments after they had given their own diagnosis:

> Dr G: I am, I must admit, concerned that she's not
> walking. She's beyond the age where she should
> be walking, and she's not talking as well as she
> should. I'm inclined to think there's a general
> delay here. How do you think she compares with
> other children?
>
> Mother: I still feel she's more easily tired than other
> children are. But she seems quite good with
> her hands.

The mother talks about other things and the doctor asks
the child to look at a book which they all watch. Eventually he comments.

> Dr G: You see, I'm not ... well, certainly I'm not
> saying she's seriously backward.
>
> Mother: No.
>
> Dr G: She seems interested and alert but she is a
> little behind. At her age one can't say what
> will happen. (The doctor elaborates.)
>
> Mother: But she is bright at play. She has a ball she
> likes, she plays with that very well.
>
> Father: And, when you take off her clothes, she recog-
> nizes all of them and the order that they
> should come off in. She knows that.
>
> Mother: Yes. What about her feet?
>
> Dr G: You know, I don't think there's much wrong there.
> I'm sure it's not her feet. (He gets parents to
> walk child.) Yes, she's using her legs a bit but
> she hasn't got her balance.
>
> Father: No. She's not got her balance.
>
> Dr G: No.
>
> Mother: She has come on slower than average.
>
> Dr G: Yes. She's coming on but just at the rate of
> slower than average. I don't know whether she'll
> speed up or not.

Although this too represents a search for agreement,
this quotation has several important differences from
those cited in the cases where a doctor was normalizing a
child. There is no assumption of an immediate and easy

concord but instead a careful discussion of the evidence,
conducted in a relatively unhurried fashion, whereas the
search and destroy method was used with speed and vigour.
When parental doubts were to be amplified rather than
dismissed doctors proceeded more slowly and indirectly.
Dr G did not repeatedly probe the parents about their
doubts or worries, he merely asked them a question which
might lead to such talk, as might his own statements and
the various demonstrations he provided, such as the book
and the walking. Doubts and their discussion were allowed
to develop gently over. time. Thus, although agreement was
certainly a high priority for staff, search is perhaps too
active a word to describe their method in such cases.
Agreement here was stalked rather than sought after;
doctors lay in wait and watched, and the end was no sudden
spring but a gradual luring towards acceptance.

For what was at issue was the parents' whole conception
of the child: its present, its future and their own
future as well. And, whereas normalizing a child might be
done in a session, as might the revelation of minor
illness, stigmatizing a child could take many months or
even years. Although it is conventional to refer to the
telling of bad news as something that occurs at one point
in time - 'When they told me' - such a description does
not capture the complex nature of the process by which
such news was broken here. To some extent this depended
on clinical uncertainty. As doctors saw a child over
time, so they gained a more accurate version of the
child's condition and capacities. Just as crucially,
however, the stages depended on the doctors' belief that
bad news should be broken slowly, that parents had to
prepare themselves for the worst, that they could not take
everything in at once, and that the news staff had to tell
should match parents' expectations:

> Dr J: She's a very nice mother. I think what we're
> trying to do is to introduce her very gradually
> to the fact that the child is very small, though
> we know she will look like a circus dwarf. You
> know the sort of child I mean? Well, we haven't
> really told the mother that. We've just said
> that she's going to be very small. Anyway, she
> seems to be a candidate for delayed development
> and there's also this increased intra-cranial
> pressure, that's going to be a problem. Now at
> six months I saw her, that was at the special
> nursery follow-up clinic and she had a head-lag
> there, but of course then it wasn't necessarily
> developmental delay. So we saw her again at

eight months, and by then she had got some head
control but she hadn't her setting balance. She
had some hand movements and was vocalizing all
right. So that seemed to be on the credit side.
But at ten months we found that she wasn't
sitting. The mother feels that otherwise she's
doing all right there. She's not a very bright
thing but I think in this case she's a pretty
good judge of what the situation is. Then she
was referred here. There has been this query
about brain damage but we've not mentioned any
of this to the mother. In fact the child had
this very bashed-about head, she looked really
awful when she was born.

The breaking of bad news was therefore an extremely
delicate operation, in which staff probed to see how much
parents suspected; produced some information and saw how
they reacted; elaborated if they were challenged; withdrew slightly if the parents looked angry, and so on.
Staff played a waiting game, not enforcing their own
definition of a child but always leaving a part to be
negotiated in each consultation, trying to build on last
time's definition, but first waiting to see how parents
commented on what had happened in the intervening weeks or
months. As far as the two can be separated, the movement
was from diagnosis to prognosis, first indicating what the
child was and then saying what it would be. The movement
from one to the other varied with the parents' receptive-
ness. No parent was told everything immediately, but some
achieved detailed and dispassionate discussion far more
quickly than others. The following example indicates both
the difficulties that might be faced and the way these
were surmounted by making little agreements at each stage.
The excerpts are from three consecutive consultations.
  This was the child's first visit to the neurological
clinic. He was four months old at this point and had
already been seen three times at the special nursery
follow-up clinic. The mother had several other children,
was highly competent and had made detailed comments on
some of her child's problems. She had not however noticed
the more serious ones, the child's spasticity and microcephaly. In his summary, the doctor started out by appealing to the shared agreement on the child's delay and
then moved on to his own diagnosis. But this was phrased
tentatively and the entire discussion of the child was in
the present not the future tense:

Dr I: He is very behind in what he's doing *of course*

(my emphasis) and although you yourself are not
very impressed with it, I think that his muscles
are rather stiff. He does have some spasticity,
this is what it's called.

Four months later, at the next visit, the mother indicated at the very beginning of the consultation that she
was sceptical if her boy had made any progress and the
doctor's own history-taking revealed very few signs of
this. This time he looked towards the future in his
summary:

> Dr I: Well, I don't find anything new. From what you
>   say he has made a very, very slight progress, not
>   very much, not very much, but a little.... I
>   hope that there will be further progress, and
>   don't be too upset if it is slow. It looks as if
>   Alan is going to be handicapped to some extent.

On the third visit, eleven months later, the mother
talked freely of the child's severe handicap: 'He's absolutely ruined.' The doctor's summary was in turn far more
specific about the future than on the previous visit.

> Dr J: He's a long way off walking now. I don't know if
>   he ever will. He's got to get sitting balance
>   first, if ... (pause) ... When he gets near
>   weight-bearing age we might ask the orthopaedic
>   surgeons if there is anything that can be done to
>   improve the mechanical performance of his feet.
>   He seems well, he's avoiding any deformities, but
>   he's certainly got quite a way to go before he's
>   got complete head control. His head is lagging
>   back a bit. The next stage after that is sitting
>   balance, he's nearly got head balance. (The
>   child is in sitting position.) How long can he
>   stay like this? Just for a few seconds?
> Mother: Yes, for a few seconds and then he keels over.
> Dr J: So we want to work on sitting balance and then
>   the next stage is weight-bearing, but he's a long
>   way off that at the moment. OK, that's fine. At
>   present you are quite happy coping with him at
>   home?
> Mother: Oh, yes (cheerfully).

Even at this stage some matters went undiscussed. The
doctor did not press the mother on her ability to cope,
though privately he felt her to be unrealistic. Further,
the full extent of the child's handicap had not yet been

revealed. The microcephaly had not been mentioned nor, as
can be seen, was any detailed statement made about the
child's mental abilities. Although the mother defined the
child as 'ruined' at one stage in the conversation, she
was eager to try and bring him on. Such eagerness was
treated as laudable but unrealistic, and an indicator that
she had still not grasped the true nature of her son's
injuries. More detailed discussion was thus postponed
until the mother herself clearly accepted such facts;
that is, until a 'reasonable' discussion of the child was
possible and reasoned agreement could be reached. Parents
and staff preserved their alliance and its rational form
by seeking agreement only when this could readily be made.

MORAL CHARACTER AND THE ALLIANCE - AN EXCEPTION

One partial exception should be made to two of the rules
that I have described in the last three chapters. I
started out by emphasizing that, no matter what a mother's
actual qualities, staff treated her as ideal. This
principle led to the further rule that whereas staff could
not criticize parents, parents could criticize staff, for
they were clients who had rights to question the service
they received. It should, however, be noted that two
mothers, whom staff privately felt to be a danger to their
child, did in fact lose some of their rights as clients.
Their moral character was not directly impugned, but they
were not allowed to criticize or object in quite the same
fashion as other mothers. In the following instance, the
mother, who had been brought to the clinic by a health
visitor and adopted a sullen attitude throughout, started
to criticize the hospital:

> Mother: He got that (scabies) when he was in hospital.
> Dr I: (rather sharply) I don't want to allocate blame.

Here the doctor felt strongly that the mother was responsible for the scabies but refrained from saying so.
She was also suspected of severe neglect, even perhaps
assault. As his remark indicated, she retained her good
character only so long as she did not impugn that of
others. Similarly, such mothers could lose their normal
rights to question or object to what was done with their
child. Here is a quotation from the second case, which
involved a mother who readily admitted that she could not
cope with her child. The child was already partly in
care, but the mother objected most strongly to the new
arrangements that were suggested. Beyond a certain point

the doctor ceased to reason with her; she was treated as
lacking the ordinary rights to object and was spoken to in
a far more authoritarian fashion than other mothers:

> Dr J: I've just been on the phone to the social work
>   department. What's been the problem?
> Mother: Well, she attacked her sister and grandfather
>   and she was throwing things - like kitchen
>   things and ornaments. She's knocked the
>   windows out and she's had two fits since I
>   last saw you.
> Dr J: Well, why did she do it? She knows she mustn't.
> Mother: Well, I smacked her then she went quiet, then
>   suddenly it all came out. I had to kick her
>   to get her off her sister when she was mad.
> Dr J: Well, there doesn't seem to be any medical
>   problem apart from these turns that she's been
>   having. Now there's been a case conference and
>   they decided that really what she needed was day
>   care. They discussed where she might get it but
>   there was no firm conclusion. Craiglee was felt
>   to be inappropriate (the child attends this
>   during the week at present), except that the
>   housemother has a very good relationship with
>   her.
> Mother: Yes, she has.
> Dr J: But sometimes they're not going to be able to
>   accommodate her and then day-fostering....
> Mother: (very sharply) No, I *won't* accept that.
> Dr J: Well, you'll have to accept one or some other.
>   (The doctor mentions a nursery as another possi-
>   bility. The mother raises transport difficul-
>   ties. From now on the doctor was distinctly curt
>   in tone with the mother, for example:) But are
>   you interested?
> Mother: Well....
> Dr J: Well, *are you interested?*

Kicking the child was not treated as an overt issue,
but such behaviour provided a covert warrant for the
removal of the mother's normal rights to question staff's
decisions. The mother was still offered a choice but her
rights to refuse it were shown to be limited, by turn of
phrase and by tone of voice, if not directly. Such
parents were expected to come quietly. The rule of reason
still applied, in that they were reasoned with and not
shouted at, but they themselves were not allowed to shout.
Thus, although parents were allies, certain rules had a
higher priority than others. All mothers were naturally
good, not all had quite the same rights to criticism.

6 Medical control

One further element in the theatre of the clinic must be considered before we go backstage and examine those more covert activities and sentiments which the bureaucratic format concealed. So far I have depicted the masks of the players and sketched in the broad themes of their relationship. Yet one quite central feature of the drama has gone largely unremarked. I have noted how parents, though allies, were nevertheless excluded from the medical college and cast as subordinates. What I have not shown is the extent to which that subordination was manifested within the various activities which made up a consultation. Put another way, we must distinguish between those matters which pertain to actors' overall status within a relationship and those rules which govern their actual participation within the action. The two are clearly related but the one does not follow directly from the other. In some encounters the lowly may be granted considerable speaking parts, while in others their baseness may be reflected both in their exclusion from large areas of the action, and in a heavy control upon those parts which they do get to play.

Here parents were both excluded and controlled. They might be partners but they were not equals, and the imbalance of power within the bureaucratic format was one of its most striking features. Although parents had some rights to question and to criticize they could use these only within an overall context of medical dominance. The technical authority given to doctors was matched by an equivalent authority to control almost every aspect of the consultations' shape, sequence and timing.

My emphasis on medical control should not be taken to mean that parents had no power to negotiate with staff. As other work has clearly shown, there are various ways in which patients may influence the course of action within

consultations (Roth, 1963; Stimson and Webb, 1975). However, although we still need to know more about such
influence, its effect should not be exaggerated. (1)
Within the bureaucratic format, and indeed within all of
the formats discussed here, medical control of the consultation was systematic, all-pervasive and almost unquestioned. Although various writers have commented on
this control (Johnson, 1972; Byrne and Long, 1976), not
all of its features have been explored; and it is such
exploration that is the aim of this chapter.

OBJECTS OF INVOLVEMENT

The medium through which control of the nuts and bolts of
interaction is exerted is the same as that used to create
the rest of a format. Selective attention is the basis on
which the whole of these little worlds rest, and participation within them is a matter of what may be defined as
relevant for whom. Thus one of the central matters
governed by the ceremonial order is the allocation of
'objects of involvement'. To put this less formally,
encounters may involve a variety of activities apart from
talk, but rights to involvement in these may not be distributed equally. We have already seen how children were
typically excluded from many areas of the medical consultation. A similar, if less extreme, exclusion applied to
their parents. Whereas doctors had rights to engage in a
wide variety of actions, parents' rights were singularly
limited.
    In clinics, doctors might do many things. They could
break off conversation with a mother to read or write a
note, or to look at the child, or to ask the nurse a
question, or to teach a student. They were also allowed
to be 'away' for long periods. Some doctors spent considerable time lost in thought, their eyes unfocussed or
their fingers drumming. They therefore had a wide variety
of sources of involvement within the consultation, and
parents typically recognized the legitimacy of such
engagement by not 'interrupting' doctors when they were
so involved. By contrast, parents had no such rights to
other activities but maintained themselves in a state of
permanent alertness during gaps in the conversation.
While the doctor read or wrote mothers waited, ready to
spring into conversation when requested to do so. They
did not read, smoke or suck sweets; and talk with their
children or their husband was strictly subordinate or, in
Goffman's terms (1972), a 'side-involvement'. Many
mothers abstained from discussion altogether, particularly

with older children.   Only if a doctor left the room might
a conversation of any normal volume or gesture begin.

Given this suppression of other involvements, it could
not be said that staff interrupted parents when they took
up their conversation once more, for there was nothing of
any substance to be interrupted.   Parents were at the
doctors' disposal, and talk could begin or end at any time
of the doctors' choosing and typically without any need
for permission or apology.

The way in which parents were allocated and accepted a
dependent role within the consultation can also be illustrated by the highly restricted set of bodily actions in
which they engaged.   Staff could move freely around the
room: now standing up;   now sitting down;   now looking
at this;   now doing that;   but parents sat in the chairs
provided for them and did not move from these except to
facilitate medical examination.   The one mother who, of
her own accord, left her chair and walked round to the
doctor's side of the desk was greeted with immense surprise.   Some parents even seemed unsure as to how far they
could make themselves comfortable.   Parents who arrived in
overcoats often sweltered in the heated rooms rather than
remove them, and one mother who arrived in a thunderstorm
sat there and dripped until the doctor asked if she wanted
to remove her coat.

Three alternative objects of medical involvement need a
further consideration.   The first of these, the discussion
of medical matters with an audience of colleagues and
students, has already been noted in the previous chapter.
There I emphasized the way in which such discussion was
overtly subordinated to the consultation between doctor
and parents.   Nevertheless, staff's ability to talk with
an audience was an important assertion of their power, for
such rights were not symmetrical.   Some parents talked at
nurses and other staff as well as to the doctor, but no
one except the doctor normally responded and such communication disappeared into a void.   By contrast, staff's
right to engage in discussion with others could be used to
influence directly their relationship with the parents.
In the following instance, the doctor used the researcher
to help to pacify a recalcitrant mother who had made a
series of complaints in a rather aggressive tone:

Dr F: Apart from her food, are there any problems?
Mother: Well, there's her sleeping.
Dr F: Well, what, doesn't she sleep?
Mother: (firmly) Well, she does now because she gets
             something to make her sleep.

Dr F grins at the baby and dangles his stethoscope in
front of it. He then says to the researcher:

> Dr F: Isn't it marvellous having a baby like this?
> (Researcher smiles. Mother smiles back at re-
> searcher.) But it's not always marvellous.
> What's this about her not sleeping?

This use of an audience was exceptional. Nevertheless,
it illustrates a potential resource that was always legitimately available to the doctor but was rather more
dubious if parents attempted it. Including the audience
in their remarks was one thing, manipulating them another.
     Besides, such manipulation was normally a most diffi-
cult task, for the audience was on the doctors' side and
could not be used against them - or so parents seemed to
assume, for in none of the consultations which used the
bureaucratic format did parents make any direct appeal to
others to intervene on their behalf. By contrast, this
happened in three out of the fifteen cases in the charity
format, and in two of these a nurse actually stepped in to
aid the mother: in the case of nappy rash cited earlier,
the nurse joined in to say that she too was guilty, that
she had always washed her babies' nappies in Ivory Snow
and had not known of its inadequacy.
     The doctors' power in the bureaucratic format was
therefore reinforced by their access to an audience which
acquiesced in their handling of the occasion and could be
manipulated to further their own ends, a resource which
was not available in quite the same manner to the parents.
(2)
     Two further asymmetries also had important consequences
for medical control. The first of these involved
children. I have already noted that children were treated
as mere side-involvements for parents. Staff's authority
extended, temporarily at least, to the relationship
between parent and child and not just to that between
parent and doctor. Indeed, the maintenance of their
authority depended on a rigid segregation of parent and
child. Staff might interact with the children whenever
they chose but parents could not do so. Staff might
switch openly between the two; parents must attend to
whatever they were bid. Staff might address parents
through the child, but they themselves were only to be
spoken to directly. Where parents' presence was deemed
to affect the relationship between staff and child too
greatly, parents were removed from the setting. After
the initial visit, both occupational and physiotherapy
staff in the Scottish hospital did not permit parents to

be present during treatment. Staff were also in charge
of the allocation of praise and blame for the child's
performance. Further, even though parents might normally
be considered to have the most extensive knowledge of
their child and to be the best interpreter of their words,
actions and feelings, such knowledge was treated as
partial and as able to be overridden where staff saw fit.

When doctors did interact with children, it was
parents' duty to assist staff in their management. In
this they were principally required to ensure that
children recognized staff's paramount authority; or, put
another way, they were obliged to underwrite the temporary
loss of their own control. Alongside this they were
expected to bring the child in a suitable condition for
examination or therapy and to aid during these as appropriate; to hold children when they struggled; to
encourage them when they failed to respond; and to soothe
them when they cried.

Such an alliance might seem to have imposed heavy
burdens upon parents, for they were deprived of most of
their normal rights over their child. Yet almost all were
loyal subordinates, even though co-operation was not
always easy, for their duties were ambiguous. On the one
hand their children were removed from their control, but
on the other hand they were still expected to help in
controlling them. Some did nothing at all but hovered
uncertainly near the child, some intervened occasionally
and hurriedly withdrew; others, as in the following
instance from the orthoptic clinic, saw it as their duty
to reinforce everything that staff said:

> Therapist G: Take your time.
> Mother: Take your time.
> Therapist G: This is the last one.
> Mother: This is the last one.
> Therapist G: Look at it.
> Mother: Look at it.
> Therapist G: Look properly now.
> Mother: Look properly.

Despite this partial removal of the child from their
keeping, parents had some rights here. They might still
interact with their sons and daughters even though such
action was clearly subordinate to, and in the end controlled by, medical staff.

The medical records were a very different matter. For
all practical purposes these belonged to the doctor and
not to the parents. In the American clinics parents had
a legal right to inspect their children's records, but

none was observed to ask the doctor if they too might
consult the file during the interaction. In all settings
the notes stayed with the doctors and in no sense were
they common property. Moreover, in many ways the presence
of the medical record was as essential to medical interaction as the presence of parents or children. (3) Just
as Dr J found it hard to continue where only the child's
brother accompanied him, so a consultation without a
record was a difficult task. Where the file for a particular case was not present, as when a child was attending another clinic at a similar time, doctors deferred
the case until the file had arrived. If they were forced
to carry on without it, as where records had to be ac-
quired from another hospital, they made continual mistakes. Such constant correction challenged their normal
professional ease. Proper medicine could only begin when
the file as well as the patient was present, for it
constituted an alternative biography to that available
from the parents, and one that had been medically
warranted.

Writing that biography was a medical and not a parental
task, and was one of the main tasks in the consultation.
Everything that parents said in clinics was for the
record. For them to speak was to permit their words to
be written down at the doctor's discretion. In all the
cases doctors made notes: some wrote as they went along,
pausing to do so after each question or test; others
waited until their investigation was complete; but all
devoted part of their time to writing. Indeed, where
official forms were used, writing could be as central an
activity as conversation with the parents. In particular,
discharges from the maternity hospital, adoption cases in
the general medical clinics, and developmental assessment
in the local authority and neurological clinics all
centred around the filling out of a form. Doctors and
nurses worked with the form openly displayed and ticked
off items one by one as they were covered. The presence
of the form and of an official pen hovering over it
defined the nature of the parental task: the production
of brief answers that could be filled in as quickly and
efficiently as possible. (4)

The record was not as obtrusive on those other occasions when there was no official form to be completed;
but it nevertheless played a major part in the action for
here too it constrained the speed, length and shape of
parents' answers. When asking questions of parents,
doctors would often not address them directly but simply
speak as they consulted the file or added fresh contents.
Only when presenting their conclusions did they routinely

look parents continuously in the face as they spoke.   For
attention was not guaranteed to parents.   Although they
had the right to ask questions or introduce topics of
conversation, they had no definite rights to an answer.
Doctors could demand this of parents but parents could not
do likewise, for doctors, as we have seen, had other legitimate objects of attention through which they could
ignore their remarks.   In the following instance, both the
child and the notes were preferred to the mother's
comments.   (The child was suffering from minor mental
retardation.)

> Dr G: (gives the child a ball) What's this? (The
>   child plays with it.)
> Mother: She's rather smart now she's older. She knows
>   her figures and she can write her own name now.
> Dr G: Yes, yes. (He gives the child some cubes and
>   writes a note, half-watching the child.)
> Mother: She doesn't like sitting, she always likes
>   something to do.
> Dr G: (carries on writing a note, then watches the
>   child intensively, then says) All right now ...
>   I'll have a word with Mr James to see what's
>   happening. There's no need to make an ap-
>   pointment for this clinic in the meantime.
> Mother: No.
> Dr G: All right, then, bye-bye (to child).
> Mother: Bye-bye.
> Child: Bye-bye.

Not only did doctors control the medical records and
use them to enforce their general control of the encounter, but parents rarely made or at least used any
records of their own.   There were only seven cases in
which parents brought along their own notes, and in three
of these it was the doctors who had asked the parents to
do this.   More importantly perhaps, no parent was ever
observed to make notes during a clinic. (5) Doctors wrote
down what they said but parents did not reciprocate.
Minutes of a kind were kept, but only staff made these,
stored them and had ready access to them.
Not only did staff have special rights to involve themselves in a wide variety of activities, but they also
largely controlled the overall timing of the consultation
and the scheduling of individual pieces of the action.
Thus it was staff who decided when a consultation both
began and ended: in only one case in the entire study did
a mother rather than a doctor end a consultation.   Time
was the doctors' and not the parents'   Not only did

parents have to arrange to see the doctor and not the
other way around, they might also have to wait even where
they had been given a set time. Doctors usually apolo-
gized for major delays, but parents had no right to interrupt and be seen at the time that had been formally set
aside for them. Similarly, once in the consultation it
was typically the doctors who scheduled events and not the
parents. As such it was doctors who normally made
comments like 'Right', 'Fine' and 'OK', which signalled
changes in the topic or the action.

CONTROLLING TALK

Just as doctors had special rights to engage in a variety
of activities besides talk with parents, and could also
largely determine the sequence and timing of those activities, so too they exerted a major control over talk
itself. In considering that control three points need
particular emphasis. The first of these is the general
absence of small talk from consultations. When staff
talked to children all kinds of personal matters might be
discussed: their school, Christmas presents, holidays or
favourite television programmes. By contrast, conversation with parents was all of a piece. Normally the
participants talked of nothing besides medical matters
either before, during or after the consultation; with
doctors there was no pre- or post-activity talk. (6)
Parents were ready to start as soon as they entered; and
as soon as they entered doctors started. Doctors opened
the talk and almost always did so with a remark that
initiated medical action. With new patients they asked
them what the problem was; with old patients they commonly inquired, 'How are things?' or 'How have you been?'
Remarks such as these might in other contexts be taken as
a general inquiry or as an occasion for talk about the
weather, their jobs, or whatever parents wished. Here,
however, 'things' meant the child's problem, and was invariably taken to be so. Such questions constituted an
opening which initiated the activity, they were not a
prelude to it. Similarly the ending of medical activity
was also the ending of talk. Once doctors had either
discharged the patient or fixed a new appointment,
patients left the room.
   Not only was talk confined almost exclusively to medical matters, it was also largely question-and-answer talk,
and rights within this were unequally distributed.
Doctors by and large asked the questions; parents did the
answering. On some occasions, after breaking bad news,

doctors did ask parents to bring a list of questions next
time. But to do so was to recognize that typically it was
they who asked the questions and not the other way round.
Parents did get some chance to ask questions but it was at
the end of the consultations, after doctors had asked
theirs.

The questions that doctors asked were also of a
distinct type. In his analysis of conversation in psychotherapy, Blum (1970) distinguishes two kinds of question
and answer talk. In the kind that is special to such occasions, the therapists' questions are to be heard simply
as occasions for general talk. Simple 'answers' are not
wanted, for the therapist is concerned with making infer-
ences about the patient's 'mind' and this requires some
display of that entity. By contrast, the questions which
were asked in the children's clinic were typically
requests for specific information and not a warrant for
general discussion. The majority of parents' answers were
therefore brief and to the point. Here, for example, is a
quotation from a developmental assessment case in a
Scottish local authority clinic:

> Dr A: Is he eating and sleeping all right?
> Mother: Yes.
> Dr A: Now, when I saw him last his eyes were a bit
>   watery, weren't they?
> Mother: Oh, they're fine now.
> Dr A: Right. Now, was the pregnancy all right?
> Mother: Yes.
> Dr A: There were no troubles during it? No kidney
>   troubles or anything?
> Mother: No.
> Dr A: It was a normal delivery, no forceps?
> Mother: No.

The third major feature of clinic talk, apart from its
specificity and its concentration on medical matters, was
the 'hidden agenda' (Scheff, 1968) to which that talk was
directed. Doctors asked for information but they did not
normally explain why they needed it, nor did they reveal
the criteria by which they judged its relevance. Some
doctors might give a brief resumé of their thinking when
they produced their conclusions, but no one gave this at
the beginning of the consultation or during the actual
questioning. Doctors had parents' answers at their own
disposal and could do with them as they wished. They
could accept them and pass on to something else, as in
the above quotation, or they might make demands for
greater precision and even on occasion check this out
with the child:

Dr G: And there's no question of his inhaling or
      swallowing anything that afternoon?
Mother: No, he didn't have anything in his mouth.
Dr G: (to child) You're quite sure, Arthur, that you
      didn't have anything in your mouth and you hadn't
      swallowed anything?
Child: No.

Similarly, where a doctor was not happy with an answer
he might continue to ask the same question until he was
satisfied. In the next example the doctor asked the
mother to describe a typical attack, but she talked
instead of a particular one. Only when he had repeated
his request three times did she rearrange the way she told
her story and start to use the general present rather than
the past particular tense:

Dr H: Now, tell me about a typical attack of sore
      tummy? What does he do?
Mother: Well, eh ... In October he had an attack ...
      he was off school for a week with the sickness
      and then he was sick again.
Dr H: Is this the typical time off for an attack? Is
      it a normal one? Is he off for a week usually?
Mother: Well, um, not usually, but that was in October.
Dr H: Will you tell me what a normal one consists of?
Mother: Well, in the winter he had two attacks, there
      was three months between them.
Dr H: Uh-huh, ummm. What's the first thing that goes
      wrong?
Mother: He complained of being sick that time, it was
      just starting up.
Dr H: Yes. Is there any pain in his tummy? Does this
      occur?
Mother: Aye, there's this pain in his tummy.
Dr H: And does this pain happen before he vomits?
Mother: I think so, and then he just, there's the pain
      and then he's sick, or sometimes it's just the
      pain.

Just as doctors repeated their questions until they got
what they wanted, they also ignored things that they took
to be irrelevant and might even interrupt a reply to ask
about the matters that really concerned them:

Dr F: Can he drink from a cup?
Mother: Yes. He's still got a bottle but....
Dr F: Can he hold a cup?
Mother: Yes, he can manage to hold one.

Not only could doctors make whatever they liked of
answers to their questions since their agenda was largely
concealed, but they also used that agenda in an extremely
rapid and routinized fashion. Such routinization was most
obvious when doctors worked from an official form, but it
was equally true of other cases. Each doctor had set
methods for handling the kinds of case which he saw and
used the same questions and the same formulations, in much
the same order, in case after case of any particular type.
(7) Thus, although parents were given opportunities to
talk they could do so only within a systematic framework
laid down by the doctor, a grid that was in daily professional use but in which they themselves had little
practice.

CONTROLLING TOPICS

As we have seen, doctors controlled the action in clinics
by limiting the amount and kind of attention they were
prepared to give to parents. Not only could they direct
the conversation but they alone had the right to engage
fully and openly in other activities outside that conversation. The right to control the consultation in this
fashion was also used to restrict the topics of consultation even more narrowly than has hitherto been mentioned. Clinic action was not only exclusively medical, but
also the medical remit was overtly defined in a most
limited fashion. Staff focussed on the individual case
and, within this, on the current physical problems which
that case involved. Only in exceptional instances was
this focus broadened.
    Take first the individualizing tendency of medical
work. I noted earlier how in any one consultation staff
concentrated on that particular child as if it constituted
a world in itself and was not just another example of X or
Y. In doing so they avoided the twin dangers of treating
the child as either mere work or just clinical material.
At the same time this focus also prevented parents from
gaining general knowledge about medicine and its ways, and
those few parents who dared to seek this were actively
discouraged. Take for instance this example from the
maternity hospital ward-round:

    Mother: Why do they measure the baby's length?
    Dr K: Well, we measure all children as it is related to
          their adult height. You probably wouldn't be
          interested.
    Mother: (eagerly) Oh, yes, I'm fascinated by all the

> things you do, but I just wondered why you were
> doing it. I must have been about four inches
> long at birth. I'm so small.
>
> Dr K: How tall is your husband?
> Mother: 5 feet 10 inches.
> Dr K: (tells the mother the average length of children
>   at birth and adds) There's not much variation in
>   this. (The mother smiles eagerly again and looks
>   as if she wants to continue the conversation, but
>   the doctor turns to talk to a registrar.)

Besides the omission of general discussion about medical matters, the range of topics covered was highly restricted. Fundamentally, doctors were only interested in
problems. Let us re-consider the quotation from Dr A's
clinic which is cited earlier in this chapter, a quotation
which is typical of interaction in almost any clinic. The
key words and phrases that recur in each interchange are
'all right', 'fine', 'no troubles' and 'normal'. As soon
as normality was established the doctor passed on to the
next topic. If there was no problem there was nothing to
talk about. Indeed, where the doctor was rushed this
might constitute the end of the interaction. Here, for
example, are two fairly typical consultations with old
patients on the maternity hospital ward-round:

> Dr K: Hello, Mrs Jones.
> Mother: Hello.
> Dr K: Is baby feeding OK?
> Mother: Yes.
> Dr K: Fine.... No problems?
> Mother: No.
> Dr K: Super.

We move on to the next bed.

> Dr K: Hello. You're an experienced mother, aren't you?
>   No problems here?
> Mother: No.
> Dr K: Fine.

We pass on to the next bed.
    Not only were doctors interested solely in problems,
but their definition of the problematic was severely
limited. This had several aspects. Let us start with
child development. This was a matter of major concern in
all the clinics, and all the doctors and therapists had
some training in the matter. However, staff only took
notice of those who were retarded. Although local au-

thority clinic doctors graded the children that they assessed, parents were not normally informed of the grade. Indeed, the fact that the child was being assessed was not normally mentioned. Only where a child was delayed were mothers told the result of the assessment.

Similarly, in all clinics mothers of delayed or handicapped children were routinely given advice on how to aid their child, but no such advice was given where babies were judged to be normal. Children, it seemed, needed to be 'brought on' only if they were 'behind'. This is not to say that doctors assumed that normal babies could not be aided in this fashion. Mothers whose babies were exceptionally competent sometimes received lavish praise by local authority doctors after they had left, but such praise was not given during the clinic, nor was criticism or advice offered where a baby was merely average. Mothers of normal children who tried to discuss the child's development in detail, and who asked about the stages at which children did this or that, were treated as 'worriers'.

Similarly, doctors normally showed little interest in the everyday difficulties posed by children. As children grew they created all kinds of new problems for their care and management. Outside clinics, among mothers waiting in the corridor, such problems were a standard topic. 'Mother-craft' was however normally excluded from clinic conversation, even where the doctor felt the mother to be relatively incompetent. This was simply not the doctor's business, it did not fall within their remit and therefore it was not dealt with. Only where it was sufficient to cause a 'medical' problem, for example severe nappy rash, was it raised, and even here its handling was often delegated to others such as health visitors or nurses.

Psychiatric matters were another topic that was normally excluded from paediatric consultations within the bureaucratic format. The avoidance of this area has already been considered in my discussion of parental character. It is worth noting here that almost all emotional issues were side-stepped and not just those which involved possible psychiatric disturbance. Clinics were not bereft of every emotion, some indeed were marked by jollity, but the emotional range was a foreshortened one. It ran simply from joy to neutrality. Where the occasion was a happy one both parties might express happiness; where it was not then by and large they expressed nothing. Here as elsewhere doctors set the tone. As we have seen, parents who tried to import a language and emotional tone appropriate to other and more cheerful occasions by laughing or displaying great affection for

their child often failed. Staff reciprocated in this
manner only when they felt it appropriate. Developmental
testing on a normal child was accompanied by all kinds of
congratulatory remarks from staff. Bad performance
received no comment. Apparent exceptions to this rule of
a limited emotional range in fact exemplify it. Staff
used dramatic language about conditions only when these
were easily remedied. Here, for example, are two doctors'
remarks to mothers on the maternity hospital ward-round:

> Dr K: Oh, what a nasty septic spot! I think that had
>   better be punctured. We'll take it through to
>   the nursery and do it there.

> Dr L: (to a nurse) Could you get this (sticky eyes)
>   seen to right away as it is rather nasty.

Serious conditions were examined without any such
comment to the parents and, just as doctors refrained from
using dramatic language, so too did almost all parents.
Clinics, it seemed, were not places for emotional display.
Bad news was broken in a matter-of-fact way and received
in much the same fashion. Doctors indicated the tragic
nature of events only by indirect means. Some, for
instance, used a quieter and more intimate tone of voice.
Some parents likewise lowered their eyes, looked embarrassed and said little or nothing, but almost none
displayed any open signs of grief. Only three parents in
all were observed to cry and then only briefly. This does
not mean that others felt no such emotions, but that
clinics were inappropriate places to express these:

> Dr J: I think they often express some of their emotions
>   as soon as they get outside the room. If I go
>   out to get something or to test the urine of the
>   next patient I find them in tears in the corri-
>   dor, when they would seem nowhere near tears in
>   the room.... They demonstrate relatively little
>   in clinic. I'm sure the picture they present at
>   home or on the bus on the way back is quite
>   different.

The absence of open grief in clinics seems linked to
the absence of any occasion formally provided for its
expression. In Sudnow's (1967) study of dying in hospitals, he noted how, when doctors broke news of a patient's
death to their relatives, they paused briefly to allow an
expression of grief. Not all relatives in fact displayed
such emotions, but all were allowed an opportunity to do

so. However, when bad news was broken in the paediatric
consultations no such opportunity was provided for parents
nor did they seem to expect this. (8) Having revealed the
existence of a serious condition, doctors simply moved on
to a discussion of further visits and possible treatment.

Such absence of occasions for grief did not mean that
staff were annoyed when it was displayed, for they saw
tears as 'natural' and as 'one end of the continuum'.
However, they acted as if those who were on the brink of
tears would rather not cry if this could be avoided. They
therefore carried on with their normal routine, or else,
when this became impossible, paused to allow parents a
chance to master their emotions. Here is the end of a
case in which the doctor had broken the news that a child
was very severely handicapped. Up to this point the
mother had been fully in control of herself; indeed she
had taken a lead in identifying problematic features about
her baby:

> Mother: Of course, if there is anything that could be
> done you would let me know?
> Dr I: Yes, of course. I don't think I'm telling you
> anything that you don't know already.
> Mother: Yes, and you would let me know if there was
> anything that could be done? You would let
> me know? (As she says this the mother becomes
> very red in the face, her eyes begin to glisten
> and she has difficulty in getting her words
> out. The doctor pauses and says nothing.
> Eventually the mother masters herself and asks
> a further question.) And when do I come back?
> Dr I: In six months' time, and you'll be seen once a
> week in physiotherapy, and otherwise I'll see
> you in six months' time.

Grief then was treated as a private matter by both
sides and not something that was appropriately expressed
in clinics. Even when mothers did cry their tears were
their own affair. The action might pause to allow them
to recover, but sorrow was not itself a topic. Doctors
did not put their arms round parents in such circumstances, nor did they encourage them to express their
feelings further. The most that any doctor did was to
murmur softly, 'I know, I know'. These matters were not
entirely neglected, for staff did act where they were
particularly worried about parents' reactions; but these
were dealt with, not in the clinic, but delegated to other
specialists such as social workers.

Not only did staff focus solely on the strictly medical

problems of a particular child, but those problems had to
be current ones, problems that were of immediate import.
Consider this apology made by the mother of a severely
handicapped child as she entered the neurological clinic:

> Mother: I feel I'm here under false pretences. I
> called in at the desk to see if I could have a
> word with you and they said, 'Come in', and
> they gave me an appointment. There's nothing
> wrong.

To arrive at a clinic without a current problem, unless
one's child was there for screening, was to lack any
proper reason for being there.

CHANGING THE RULES

There is one final aspect of the medical control of these
consultations that requires mention, although it need only
be brief since I have touched upon it several times in the
preceding chapters.

Far from being immutable, the bureaucratic format could
itself be modified when the occasion arose, and the right
to control such alteration formed a crucial part of the
doctors' armoury. There were basically two kinds of
changes that might be made in the rules. The first and
most fundamental of these was to shift the entire format
and substitute another, or at least blend in elements of
two formats into the same encounter. As we shall see
later, doctors were not entirely free agents in this
respect; nevertheless it was they who chose when to admit
parents to a collegial discussion and not the parents
themselves; and it was largely up to doctors to decide
how far a clinical discussion with other staff or students
might be permitted. The occasional parent might try to
enforce the conventions of the private format but, unless
they were also paying for the service, such attempts did
not succeed.

The fact that the format was in some sense at the
doctor's disposal was one of the principal constraints
upon parental criticism or complaint. To step too far out
of line might produce a change to another and far less
pleasant ceremonial order. No such complete switch was
actually observed, although doctors hinted at its possibility in censuring mothers of revealed bad character.
Nevertheless it remained a permanent possibility and one
that is certainly exercised in other kinds of medical
setting, as will be seen later.

The second right which doctors had in this respect was
to modify one or two of the rules while still retaining
the overall form of the bureaucratic mode. Two good
examples of this procedure have already been given.
Parents were normally cast as technically incompetent but,
where it suited doctors' purposes, as when they wished to
normalize or to stigmatize a child, they might be granted
a temporary equality - so long at least as they supported
the doctor's own judgment. This right to confer identities upon the other participants, or the privilege of
'alter-casting' in Weinstein's (1966) phrase, was also
seen in the removal from two mothers of the normal parental rights to criticism.

    But other sorts of rule might be modified as well.
Indeed in some therapy sessions the heavy control of
conversation was so relaxed that the ceremonial order no
longer resembled the bureaucratic format. What happened
on such occasions is nevertheless worth a brief inspection
since the contrast may still tell us something about the
normal mode. We must also examine the somewhat lesser
relaxation of control that could occur with the parents of
severely handicapped children, for such instances formed
the major, though only partial, exception to the rule of
doctor domination of the proceedings.

SPECIAL CASES - THERAPY

In two of the settings where therapy was done - the occupational and physiotherapy departments of the Scottish
hospital - parents were excluded from the treatment
sessions and were seen, usually briefly, before and after
each session. Compared with medical consultations in
clinics, such meetings were casual and relatively easy
affairs. This was partly due to the therapists' status.
They too were women, while they had no formal responsibility for assessing a child's condition, or for informing
mothers about it. They were also much lower in the hospital hierarchy than doctors, and for some of them, their
social origins were rather nearer those of the majority
of patients. Moreover, although they routinely discussed
the child's performance in therapy, such discussion typically lacked a heavily controlled agenda. Indeed, other
identities besides those of therapist and parent were used
to generate topics of conversation. A discussion of the
child's performance could on occasion be followed by all
manner of general topics which had little to do with
therapy. Since they saw parents so often, usually either
weekly or fortnightly, and over such a long period - often

several years - therapists could become part of the
routine life of parent and child. As such they might
acquire details of the parents' interests, mood, holidays,
home and work. While doctors had no time in which to get
to know a child, therapists' whole management technique
was based upon such knowledge. For some children, therapists - like teachers - became central figures in their
lives, and their mothers commented on how they looked
forward to therapy and on what they had said about it last
time. Finally, whereas clinic visits were infrequent, the
weekly visits to therapy corresponded to the parents' own
time-scale and to their everyday perception of change in
the child.

All this meant that each side could take so much more
for granted, both about each other and about the child,
than was possible in clinic consultations. Whereas for
doctors most children were part of an undifferentiated
mass, to and about whom they could say little more than
repeat the standard adult formulae used to inquire of the
young, therapists could display a rich store of personal
information about each patient. As such, mothers could
simply assume that their child was well known to the
therapist, they did not have to explain, merely allude.
Since meetings were frequent both sides could raise
matters as they arose and when they felt the time was
right. Topics could flow 'naturally' out of the conversation and did not have to be openly enforced. This
greater ease was heightened by the absence of any overt
records or record-taking in normal conversations with
parents. Doctors pooled their records in a central system
and for them continuity resided primarily with the files
and not with their personal knowledge of the patients;
but therapists knew them from acquaintance as much as from
their notes.

Despite these differences one must not overemphasize
the contrast between doctors and therapists. The latter
did not devote much of their time to parents, for mothers
often brought and fetched their children with barely more
than a minute or two's conversation. Some mothers were
reticent and staff never got to know them, while, whatever
their relationship, therapists owed their primary al-
legiance to the hospital and not to the mothers. Although
there was often no overt agenda in their chats with
parents, in practice they were searching for information
about mothers' attitudes or family conditions and, where
relevant, this was passed to other staff. Therapists
asked mothers about their lives, mothers did not normally
respond in kind.

SPECIAL CASES - SERIOUS CONDITIONS (9)

The second exception to the principle of rigorous medical
control concerns cases that are far more central to my
analysis. Where a child was seriously and chronically ill
then medical control might be relaxed to suit the special
medical tasks which such conditions created. As we have
seen, severely handicapped children placed a major strain
upon their parents. The assessment of their ability to
cope with this burden could not be done solely by the
interrogatory style typical of more normal consultations.
For this purpose, staff used the psychotherapists' style
in addition to their usual manner and sought to produce
displays of talk as evidence of parents' frame of mind.
Such general conversation served a further goal. We have
noted how slowly doctors broke the worst news, how they
waited for signs that the mothers themselves had come to
realize the facts of their child's condition. Again, the
accurate judgment of parents' version of their children
required a more relaxed, more equal conversation than
that which was typical of less serious conditions. In
consequence, staff allowed parents rather more opportunity
to set the agenda. Mothers' interest and wonder at the
minutiae of their child's development, something which was
normally excluded from clinic interaction, might here be a
most relevant topic. In this quotation a mother talks
about her very severely handicapped son. The mother after
discussing blood tests, an EEG and the child's hearing -
all topics initiated by the doctor - introduces a topic of
her own:

>Mother: We've seen Mrs Sheila (physiotherapist) today
>and she's very pleased with him and said he was
>coming on well. She said he may be ready for
>his shoes soon. He seems to be making another
>spurt. He's altogether stronger and asserting
>his rights. For example, you can't shove food
>at him either. If he doesn't want to, then he
>won't.
>
>Dr I: He's becoming more of an individual?
>
>Mother: Yes, it's lovely to get this feeling that I
>just can't manipulate him as I want, that he's
>got his own will. I've got some exercises now
>for him from Mrs Sheila. He's splaying his
>legs out now so he can sit quite nicely. He's
>actually managing to sit on the floor by
>himself. Another problem that we had was him
>rubbing his head on the back of the settee.
>Mrs Sheila said we should stop him doing this

as it would put him back into wrong positions,
so that's sorted too.

Dr I: I get the feeling that you're reasonably pleased
with the way things are going at the moment.

Mother: Yes. Another thing is that he would never put
his arm around you when you carried him and if
he fell over he would never put his arm out to
support himself, he just squealed. But in the
last few weeks he's started to grab hold of you
and if I carry him upstairs he'll put his arm
round me. These are very small things, I
realize, but they're things he's developing
now.

Dr I: They're signs of progress, however small.

Mother: Yes, like the first time he broke a cup for me.
I was thrilled that he'd got to the stage where
he realized that if you threw something over
the side of the cot it made a nice noise. And
now he's started to have odd nocturnal dreams,
I think.

As can be seen, the doctor allowed the mother to talk
freely, not imposing his own agenda but simply repeating
what she had said in a polite fashion and allowing her to
raise fresh topics. The medical agenda might be broadened
in other ways as well. In the more serious cases where
children attended repeatedly, it was common for parents to
raise all kinds of minor medical problems which had little
or nothing to do with the main condition, or with the
doctors' specialist skill. These were dealt with cheerily
along with all the rest. Attendance at the clinic might
also be continued long after it had any real medical relevance. Thus whereas normally the agenda was highly restricted, in some cases hospital staff took on the role
of the general practitioner:

Dr I: There's no real point in some ways in still
seeing Angela but I like to, as you can't really
rely on GPs. I'm hopeless at working out which
GPs are the really good ones. The only contact
I have with them is through their letters. I
hardly ever meet any GPs in the city. Some
doctors can work it out but I can't. It takes
years to do anyway. Doctors who have been here
a very long time, like Dr Fitzsimmons and
Dr Simpson, have got to know which GPs are
reliable and obviously it helps if you've been
trained here. Dr McAllister trained here and
knows quite a few of them personally. Really,

it should be the GP's job to check up on children
like this, but as so many don't you can't rely on
it. So in the end the paediatrician has to take
on the responsibility of keeping an eye on them.

As was noted earlier, not only did paediatricians
discuss a much wider range of personal problems with the
parents of such children, but they also assumed a managerial responsibility as regards other hospital and local
authority services and checked on parents' attendance at
these and their feelings about them. This broadening of
the agenda meant that parents had rather more control over
the discussion in such cases. Once again, this point must
not be over-stressed. As we have seen, doctors were
cautious about the information they produced and shyed
away from any criticism of other services. Moreover,
although they allowed parents to talk more freely about
their children such conversation was still linked to the
doctors' agenda and took place under their control.

7 Ease and tension in the alliance

Having examined the various components which together made up the bureaucratic format, we can now step back a little and consider the overall fit between this surface ceremony and the more covert sentiments and actions of the partici- pants. The outer form in which it cast the relationship of doctors and parents was flattering, if rather tightly controlled. In a strictly technical sense the format proved most successful for, despite the extremely varied circumstances in which it was applied, it was only on quite exceptional occasions that any major modification was necessary. Another good indicator of this achievement is the way in which almost all the participants managed to contain whatever personal feelings they may have had, either about each other or about the events under con- sideration. Consultations were both formal and polite, and strong emotions were suppressed. No doctor who used the bureaucratic format was ever seen to get angry with a parent, while only a handful of parents came anywhere near anger and overtly such emotions were quickly dissipated. Similarly, despite the great tragedy that was sometimes involved, almost no one cried.

It must not be supposed that this technical success meant that all consultations were managed with equal ease. As I have emphasized, a role format is primarily a matter of surface ceremony. It is an entity to which partici- pants pay formal respect but it does not necessarily re- flect how they actually feel about events, nor is it an accurate guide to all the action within any particular encounter. Many things may be done so long as they are decently clothed. Sometimes, of course, there is a ready fit between the ceremonial order of an encounter and the wider worlds of those who act within it. On these 'easeful' (Goffman, 1961) occasions the participants may feel no sense of strain and become completely engrossed

within the action. But if there is any serious discrepancy between surface and substance, between the overt order
and the covert reality as perceived by one or all of the
participants, then such occasions are marked by a continu-
ous tension, a tension which is reflected in continual
efforts to bridge or conceal the crevasse. Since my data
is largely observational my account will focus primarily
on these visible signs of strain rather than on the
subjective accounts found in some other work (e.g.,
Stimson and Webb, 1975; Strong, 1977a).

I have, of course, already considered a wide variety of
sources of tension. However, my account has been partial
for, in seeking to show the universality of the format's
rules, I have concentrated on the especially adverse
situations and neglected those features which posed
systematic difficulties in every consultation. Up till
now it may have seemed that, where parents were relatively
competent and the child's condition amenable to medical
treatment, then the alliance could be made with great
ease. The one possibly harsh note has been the ubiquity
of medical dominance. There were, however, a number of
other, general features which were equally potent sources
of strain. Great ease was in fact a relatively rare occurrence; and the alliance, although constructed for
mothers, was, as will be seen, more suited to foster-
mothers - fellow-professionals whose knowledge and involvement more closely matched that of medical staff.

MEDICAL TIME

One major source of strain lay in the marked discrepancy
between the overt medical emphasis on service to the individual client and the actual setting and timing of that
service. Certain potentially offensive matters might be
carefully excluded; but the bureaucratic setting, and the
medical control of action within that setting, these could
not be wished away. Doctors did not see patients in their
own homes and at their own times. Instead patients waited
on doctors. To attend an outpatient clinic was to enter
an elaborate and formalized bureaucracy whose rituals had
an iconographic as well as a functional significance,
revealing both the precise nature of the doctor's time,
and that each client was simply one amongst many. Simply
to get the attention of a doctor, parents had to make a
formal appointment, for which they received a card. On
arrival at a hospital they were confronted by a large
building whose interior, though full of bustle and activity, was also permeated by a sense of seriousness and en-

forced quiet. Entrance to this, or to a city clinic, required investigation by a receptionist and after that there were still further intermediaries, nurses or health visitors in uniform, who controlled immediate access to each doctor. Time did not belong to parents but to doctors, and mothers could only be seen when staff were ready for them. Thus, even before the consultation began certain crucial features of its form were already present in embryo. Waiting for an appointment or waiting outside the clinic told parents what their status would be once they were inside.

Within this framework, the amount of time allocated to parents was both brief and bureaucratically regulated, even though doctors had some flexibility in the amount they gave to individual cases - a few patients might receive two or even three times their official allowance. But such time was bought at a cost; other patients had to receive less than their due or else doctors had to skimp other work. Further, such variation took place within very narrow limits compared to the complexity and importance of some of the issues that were addressed. Here are a doctor's comments on reading through the file of a child who had been referred to him from another clinic with suspected developmental delay. The clinic is running half an hour late.

> Dr J: I don't understand this. James was seen last
> week but none of the relevant tests have been
> done. What on earth can I do? I suppose all I
> can do is the milestones.... Oh, heavens!
> (reads out notes) 'The mother fears that there
> is a diagnosis of leukaemia which is being hidden
> from her! ... The child lives with granny and is
> best seen with the grandmother.'
> Nurse: Well, it's the mother and father that are here
> with her today.
> Dr J: Oh, no! I wonder if the mother is being upset by
> all these referrals? And it says here that I'm
> to decrease the mother's fears. In *fifteen*
> *minutes* (the time formally allotted for the
> case)!

Given such narrow limits the only feasible solution for staff was to control the nature, sequence and timing of the action as tightly as was described in the previous chapter. Exceptions were possible only for the exceptional patient. To circumscribe the consultation in this fashion had effects well beyond the rather dramatic problems of the case cited above. Things happened at the

doctor's pace and not at that of the parents. They had
little time to pause for thought or to modify a previous
answer. Since time was the doctor's they could not ask
him to slow down or request an extra ten minutes at the
end. Once topics had been dealt with they were normally
gone for ever, for it was hard to return with second and
fresher thoughts. Since time was limited and questions
were pointed, answers had to be brief. The vague and
circuitous nature of everyday talk about illness had no
place here, nor could there normally be any mention of
the ways in which that particular illness had a meaning
in parents' lives. As we have seen, how they felt about
their child, the practical problems of its condition,
their ups and downs: all of these were normally excluded.
The transaction was rapid, focussed and, above all, impersonal.

This impersonality was always a threat to the ideology
of the 'alliance', but posed a special threat to the more
long-term and serious cases. Not only was the agenda
sometimes broader here, but the regularity of parental
visits could lead to the expectation of a more personal
friendship. However, not only was there a considerable
staff turnover but also, even where the same doctor continued to treat the same patient over the years, his
recollection of the case rested as much in the records as
in his own memory. On occasion, almost everything, even
the parents' name, might be forgotten:

    Dr I: Hello. Do come in.
    Grandmother: Hello.
    Dr I: Mrs Hutchison, isn't it?
    Grandmother: Mrs Innes!
    Dr I: Mrs Innes.... Sorry! I thought I remembered it.
        She's been in for ... (pause)
    Grandmother: For therapy.
    Dr I: In the inpatients for therapy!
    Grandmother: Yes, as an inpatient.
    Dr I: She's not in Marchbanks yet?
    Grandmother: No, no. She's not in there yet. I've
                been up to see it as you suggested but
                she's got to wait for a bed. They've put
                her on the waiting list.

MEDICINE AND MORALITY

A similar discrepancy between ceremony and substance may
be found in the treatment of parents' character. The
ideal nature ascribed to parents within the bureaucratic

format was one of its most striking features. Yet to
understand fully the working of encounters within that
format one must at the same time grasp a quite opposite
proposition. Despite the surface neutrality of the ceremonial order, medical work in all these consultations
necessarily involved routine and systematic moral investigation. On the one hand doctors treated parents with the
greatest delicacy, on the other hand they covertly scrutinized their competence and character in a myriad different
ways.

The assessment of the patients' or their representatives' moral character is a central feature of medical
encounters in any kind of format. To see why this is so,
some brief remarks are necessary on the nature of medical
phenomena. In analysing any kind of event one makes use
of what Goffman (1975a, p.22) has termed 'two broad
classes of primary framework, "natural" and "social"'. In
natural frameworks, events are seen as unguided and un-
willed. Since they are purely physical and quite separate
from human action, there can be no standards of success or
failure here. By contrast, social phenomena are viewed as
aimed and controlled and are thus subject to assessment as
regards their efficiency and morality. Despite this apparently clear dichotomy, the actual application of these
frameworks is often a difficult matter, for the natural
and the social are interwoven in complex ways.

Medical matters are a good example of such complexity.
On the one hand many medical phenomena have clearly
physical causes and are treated by largely physical means.
As such, sickness often serves as a legitimate excuse. On
the other hand, illness is embodied and is thus also part
of the social world: many conditions are caused by or
partly correlated with social events, while their recognition and treatment are in many ways social phenomena, as
are many of their consequences. The investigation of
illness in any one patient is therefore as much an inquiry
into the social as into the natural sphere, and is necessarily a moral as well as a physical inquiry.

The extent to which staff, on the basis of such assessment, actually condemned parents when in private,
varied considerably. Some, as in this instance, were
forthright:

    TD: When she (social worker) first made contact there
        she really wanted to change the family, but she
        soon learnt that you couldn't. You can't change
        things with the Millers and people like them. It
        just goes on.... I've given her lots of clothes
        and things, I've really tried to help that family

> but she's just pawned them straightaway.... Her
> husband is a pig, he's a big man with pop-eyes, a
> very nasty piece of work.

Other avoided such judgments. Here another therapist
argues that one should never condemn parents:

> TE: I don't think we're here to judge the parents. I
> think that the parents, they've got that child
> twenty-four hours a day ... trying to put oneself
> into the position of having a child twenty-four
> hours a day ... I think that's what we've constant-
> ly tried to do.

But even though staff differed in the extent to which
they moralized about their clientele, all routinely engaged in social and thus ultimately moral assessment.
Some might not in fact condemn parents, but their inquiries provided the material from which indictments could
always be made.
This moral assessment had several important dimensions.
First let us consider the cause of the child's condition.
I have already touched on the possible psychiatric links
with many childhood complaints, but even in more clearly
physical ailments, parents might still be held partly responsible. The conditions in which the family lived,
their knowledge of health and diet, and the care which
mothers had taken, all played a part in the incidence of
disease. One crucial indicator of these matters, or so
staff felt, was social class; and data were gathered on
all aspects of this. Staff noted parents' accent, asked
about their occupation and examined their address with
some care:

> Dr G: They're from Danzig Terrace. That's a notorious
> place in the city for problem families.

The doctor next looks at the child's height and weight
which have been given him by a nurse.

> Dr G: Well, they're in the normal range. ... (pause)
> ... I suppose they are about average for Danzig
> Terrace.

Apart from noting such background features, staff
routinely assessed, in so far as they were able, the care
that parents gave their children. Besides considering the
extent to which parents had complied with medical advice,
routine questioning and physical examination gave them the

opportunity to note the child's general state and to check
its nourishment and cleanliness.   Indeed, this was a
mandatory part of staff's work.   Although children still
belong legally to their parents, in both Britain and the
United States the State has increasingly intervened within
the family and medical staff are crucial agents in such
intervention.   This showed itself in a number of different
ways.   In the developmental assessment carried out in the
Scottish local authority clinics, doctors were required to
grade parental care on an official form, and strong attempts were made to assess every young child in the City.
Under State law the American doctors faced legal action if
they failed to report any case where they suspected the
possibility of child abuse.   Although it was extremely
rare for children to be removed from their parents on
medical grounds, in all settings the doctors had access
to para-medical workers with both the training and the
mandate to intervene within the family.   The Scottish
local authority had large numbers of health visitors who
regularly visited all newborn babies, while both hospitals
had their own social workers who could investigate any
family matters about which doctors were worried.
    Although the threat of potential investigation hung
over every clinic, relatively few parents were in fact
investigated since most attained what doctors took to be
a reasonable, if not perfect, standard of care.   But at
the same time, however well they cared for their children,
all mothers were likely to fail on at least one central
aspect of a parent's duty.   I have noted how fathers were
openly distrusted as reliable witnesses but, although
mothers were overtly treated as fully competent in this
respect, in private doctors were sceptical:

  Dr G: The mother I think had observed them (small fits)
         in the child but just hadn't noticed them.   We're
         used to this sort of thing, but this is her first
         baby.   It shows you, you just can't rely on
         mothers knowing what to expect and what to under-
         stand from the baby's behaviour.   When we asked
         her about them she said nothing about it.

    Such scepticism about parents' ability to notice the
problematic informed whole areas of medical practice.   Developmental screening, for instance, was premised on the
assumption that parents were unable to detect many forms
of delay, at least in their early stages.   Not only did
parents not notice things that doctors defined as important, but staff also suspected the accuracy of what
they did report.   Here are Dr G's comments to the students
as he reads from a referral letter:

Dr G: 'The mother says the child has right occipital
      headaches.' Now is it likely that a five-year-
      old could say to his mother that he has a
      headache? It's very rare. It's even rarer to
      locate it. So I immediately say that this is the
      mother's interpretation.... Is it likely that a
      five-year-old would come up to his mother and
      say, 'I've got a right occipital headache'
      (laughter). So immediately one has to think
      about how reliable the mother is.

These matters were often summed up in a word. The most
common medical classification of parents was whether they
were 'bright' or 'dim'; 'intelligent' or 'unintelligent':

Registrar: The mother *claims* it's a thirty-two week
          pregnancy. She also says X.
Dr J: She doesn't sound very bright.
Registrar: She's not.

Dr Y: It sounds as if the father hasn't got two neurons
      to rub together.

Dr G: That mother's not very bright either. She says
      that she thinks that the child is going to become
      smart in time, yet there's no doubt that she'll
      be a very backward child.

The other key quality for which doctors searched was
how far parents were 'sensible'. (1) Being 'sensible'
meant putting things in their proper context; not
worrying without any cause; not letting one's emotions
influence what one reported to doctors; accepting one's
fate; and making hard decisions when these had to be
made. In other words it meant an active and competent
compliance with medical staff. While some mothers,
'worriers', saw problems where there were none, and
others tried to overcome the impossible, the ideal parent
had a nice balance of involvement and detachment, subordination and concern. Here, for example, a therapist discusses the mother of a severely handicapped child:

TE: She's marvellous. The best of them all. She's
    ever so detached and yet ever so loving and she
    genuinely wants to know what's best for her child.

Whatever parents' actual qualities, however much they
loved their children and cared for them in sensible and
intelligent ways, the routine background questioning which

was a central part of taking a history might well uncover other shameful matters that were never normally revealed. Some children were illegitimate and so, on occasion, were parents. Spouses might be separated or divorced, alcoholic or mad. Such matters were only rarely mentioned, but where they existed there was always the possibility of their discovery. Indeed, medical questioning might even reveal discrediting identities of which a parent was previously unaware. The following quotation is from the case of a boy with suspected epilepsy:

Dr I: And your husband? How old is he?
Mother: 25.
Dr I: And he's in good health?
Mother: Hmm.
Dr I: Now *he's* had some attacks, hasn't he?
Mother: Well, I don't really know. Not since we were
        married.
Dr I: Oh, Dr Martin (GP) mentions that he was in
        Benlogie Hospital (principally an institutional
        hospital for the retarded).
Mother: He was in for three years.
Dr I: You don't know what he was in there for, do you?
Mother: I don't know. He got himself into trouble.
        Stealing, I think it was.
Dr I: How old was he then, do you know?
Mother: About 16. He came out when he was 19.
Dr I: When he was 19, yes. But you....
Mother: I thought he was in for trouble.
Dr I: Uh-huh. You didn't know then that he'd had some
        attacks?
Mother: No.
Dr I: He's had some blackouts. I think your husband
        will have told Dr Martin about them. (Mother
        looks blank.) What's your husband's work?
Mother: He's in the cleansing.
Dr I: He's in the Street Cleansing Department, is he?
        Uh-huh. Did you go to an ordinary school?
Mother: Yes, an ordinary school.

Thus no matter how technical the manner in which staff asked their questions and however much they abstained from comment, medical inquiry could always be read by parents as a check on their competence and good character. Even if staff denied that assessment was being done, this offered no real guarantee:

Dr I: Are you still pumping her valve?
Mother: Yes.

Dr I: How many times a day?
Mother: *You* told me ten times.
Dr I: I'm not trying to catch you out. (Mother laughs
     disbelievingly.)

Parents' awareness of the underlying nature of consultations was shown most clearly in their appearance.
Children were scrubbed, shined and dressed in their
smartest clothes, (2) as indeed were their representatives, who often wore their best suit for the occasion.
Of course, the display of moral worth extended beyond
the matter of appropriate costume. Take the matter of
compliance with medical advice. Some parents were quick
to reveal their effort and motivation:

TG: Hello, and how's Peter?
Mother: Fine. Show Miss Carson your white patch. It
     proves you've been wearing it (she laughs).

A rather more subtle strategy can be found in another
mother's comments when she arrived to collect her child
from therapy. The mother was suspected by the therapist
of cossetting the child and carrying her rather than
making her walk:

Mother: Do you want a walk?
Child: Yes.
Mother: Thank Goodness!

Such displays of righteousness could be elicited by
almost any question; for not only were staff engaged in
covert moral judgment but the criteria which they used
were necessarily unclear to parents. This was not simply
a matter of this judgment being hidden, for the inter-
weaving of the natural and the social was ambiguous in
itself. Moreover, in a society with major ethnic, class,
occupational and religious divisions, there are a variety
of standards by which action may be judged, and the
opinions of any one person cannot be known in advance.
In the essentially middle-class setting of the hospital
clinic, working-class parents were at a particular disad-
vantage. They were often unsure of the proper behaviour
expected of a young child and controlled their offspring
with considerable severity. Middle-class parents looked
on in amused tolerance as their two-year-olds played on
the floor or interrupted the doctor, but many working-
class parents went red with embarrassment at such behaviour and were plainly worried how far it reflected on
themselves. In addition to these other uncertainties, one

must also note that parents have a great variety of responsibilities, many of which contradict each other. As
regards their child they have to care for it but yet not
spoil it and, apart from their child, they have many other
duties. They have responsibilities towards their spouses,
their own parents, their other children and towards themselves. Each of these may conflict in some way and it is
always a matter of practical judgment as to which rule
should prevail in any one instance.

As a result of all these ambiguities, parents could
never know for certain just when they were being judged
and whether or not they had passed. On one occasion or
another any medical remark might bring forth a parental
justification or display of moral concern:

Dr I: He still uses both hands?
Mother: He's left-handed. But I don't try to stop him
        being left-handed. I've left all my children
        to use whichever hand they want.

Dr F: And is she feeding herself with a spoon yet?
Mother: Well, I haven't had time for that yet.
Dr F: (to students) Well, they don't usually feed
        themselves at this stage.

Dr J: Well, she's been a model patient.
Mother: She hasn't been like this the last two or three
        times she's come. I was so ashamed of her.

Besides the considerable difficulties of managing young
children, parents faced many other problems in fulfilling
their duties towards staff. I have already discussed the
conflict between, on the one hand, the twin rules of
collegial authority and medical control and, on the other
hand, parents' own right to reasonable criticism. Several
other such conflicts must also be noted. Parents had a
right, even a duty, to raise their worries about their
child. But to do so was fraught with danger. Since most
parents were ignorant they could not always know what
would count as a proper medical problem worthy of staff's
consideration. Moreover, since fears are an emotional as
well as a rational matter and are known to be so, even
medical training gave parents no guarantee that they were
right. If there was in fact no problem, then the parents
not only wasted the doctor's time but discredited themselves. They might, perhaps, be judged as silly, needless
worriers. Even if they were correct they might still have
done something wrong. The child might have a different
problem from the one they thought it had, or else they

should have spotted it earlier, or handled it in a different way. In consequence, some parents prefaced their
worries with apologies or made disclaimers afterwards:

> Dr B: And what can we do for you, Mrs Mitchell?
> Mother: Well, I may be daft but I think he's teething.

> Dr C decides that there is no problem.
> Mother: It's just these spots.... Other people notice
>   it and.... (her voice trails off)

> Father: There is one thing. I don't know whether it's
>   relevant or not, but Michael never moved as
>   much before he was born as our earlier baby.
> Dr I: Well, some children just do move and others
>   don't.
> Father: Well, it's probably stupid of me to bring this
>   up but I just wondered.
> Dr I: Not at all.

More seriously, the possible embarrassment which such
statements portray may have deterred many parents from
raising those matters which troubled them most deeply. I
have already noted the elaborate search procedures which
were required to uncover certain parental doubts. Yet
typically these were used only when staff were certain
both that the parents were worried and also that there
were no real grounds for such worry. In other words, for
worries to be dealt with parents had normally to raise
them themselves and, as we have just seen, there were
several powerful deterrents to this.
I shall give just one example of the difficulties that
this may have caused, that of chronic handicap. In many
cases the precise cause of the condition was unknown.
Quite why a child was spastic or retarded was usually
uncertain, something which led to a good deal of parental
speculation. In discussion with students and with the
researchers doctors often mentioned this and the mistaken
theories parents often produced. They had, it would seem,
all kinds of worrying beliefs about causation, many of
which centred round personal responsibility. One mother
ascribed her child's condition to bumping into a lamp-post
when pregnant, another to hanging curtains too near term.
Yet these theories were only discussed if the parents
themselves raised them, and this applied to a strictly
limited number of cases. Most parents showed a marked
reluctance to reveal such fears and, correspondingly,
doctors seemed unwilling to explore them in any detail.
No doctor made routine inquiries into these matters and,

even when the topic was raised, it was usually dealt with
in a brisk, no-nonsense fashion that seemed unsuited to
the possible agony and embarrassment that the issue might
cause for parents.

The following instance brings out several of these
features. Quite often the matter seemed so difficult to
raise that it was fathers and not mothers who asked about
it. Here, the question is asked even more indirectly:

Dr J: Well, all seems to be going fine. I'll see her
      again in a year's time.
Mother: She's very bright, it's as if she's tired, her
      hand ... (the child is spastic).
Dr J: Yes, more than her leg.
Mother: Yes, I think she will be all right ... (pause)
      ... Shona Brown is in Jane's nursery too and
      her mother blames herself for it.
Dr J: Does she come here?
Mother: Yes, she can't work out why this happened to
      her. They said something about her heartbeat
      being down in labour.
Dr J: Well, it's very often that we can't find a reason
      for these things.
Mother: It may have been that I knocked myself when I
      was seven months pregnant.
Dr J: I shouldn't think it would have been that.
Mother: Well, the cord was trapped.
Dr J: Yes, that's more likely. Hey, she's away with my
      bricks!
Mother: Yes! (grabs child) And so we make an ap-
      pointment for a year.
Dr J: Yes, for a year. That's fine. Bye.
Mother: Bye.

This mutual difficulty derived from a combination of
factors. I have just noted the problem that these issues
created for parents, while medical avoidance of the topic
also seems based on matters treated earlier. The pressure
of time meant that staff had every incentive to ignore
anything that was not placed firmly on the agenda, while
the exploration of these matters could seriously threaten
the doctor's status. Where staff could say nothing with
any certainty, their technical authority might well be
placed in doubt. As one doctor admitted, 'You might as
well ask a man in a fairground as me, we just don't know.'

Another source of embarrassment and potential judgment
for parents lay in the distinctly positivist conception of
a parent's duties that was embodied in medical interrogation. As can be seen from staff's treatment of parents

with medical pretensions, the ideal parent did not theo-
rize about what they had observed but merely reported 'the
facts' and left the doctor to consider what these might
mean. Parents who offered their own diagnoses created yet
more work for doctors. Yet this ideal was quite unworka-
ble in practice. As Bloor and Horobin (1975) have noted,
many types of medical practice are based on the assumption
that patients or their representatives possess the ability
to diagnose that they have a medical problem. Yet, having
used their skills and made the decision to seek advice,
they are supposed to remain passive during the consultation, a situation that may often lead to conflict.
Besides this, the positivist model is internally inco-
herent. To cite a previous quotation: 'The mother I
think had observed them (fits) in the child but just
hadn't noticed them.' In other words, since the mother
lacked any proper criteria for investing medical significance in her child's behaviour, she was unable to report
on it in any fashion relevant to the doctor's purposes.
In other words, competent observation depended upon having
an appropriate theory and this was something that most
parents lacked. Even when parents attempted to stick to
'the facts', it quickly became evident that some facts,
such as teething, on which they placed great significance
were of no interest to staff, while other matters into
which they had made no inquiry themselves were probed in
great detail. Parents' inability to provide consistently
accurate or relevant information was also indicated by
doctors' recourse to competing sources of data such as
the medical record or physical examination.
    Telling a story in such circumstances could thus become
most difficult for parents. The mere fact that a doctor
asked a question might be seen as containing an implicit
assumption that any competent mother could answer it.
Moreover, just telling their story to an expert could
shake any confidence that parents might have held in it,
for it was necessarily constructed according to lay criteria, criteria of which they might only become aware when
in the presence of experts. Even if staff made no comment
on what was said, their mere presence might produce all
kinds of doubts and modifications in the stories parents
told. And if they asked about things that parents had not
thought of or ignored matters that they had taken to be
central, then any coherence of or confidence in their
story could easily disappear. In the following instance
the mother was reduced to long periods of silence:

Dr I: When did he have the first one?
Mother: He was three years old, about a year ago.

Dr I: What was it like?
Mother: His eyes roll up and he stares.
Dr I: Did he have a temperature?
Mother: Yes, and a sore throat. He went a bit rigid
the second time. (She elaborates.)
Dr I: Can we stick to the first one?

Mother stops but then continues to describe a typical
attack drawing on various attacks he has had.

Dr I: I just want to know about the first one for the
moment. (Mother stays silent.) Did he do
anything else? (Mother stays silent.) Did he
jerk or shake at all?
Mother: Yes, a bit.

Thus the idealized competence granted to mothers, the
overt assumption of their intelligence, rationality and
reliability, was potentially undercut by the most routine
of medical practices. A request for elaboration or for
rephrasing, the asking of a question, or the examination
of a file, all of these carried with them a consistent
threat to that pristine parental image that was so central
a part of the ceremonial order. Nor were these the only
risks that parents ran, for threats to their character and
competence came, as we have seen, from a wide variety of
sources. Medical work was necessarily social and thus
moral work.

AUDIENCE EFFECTS

A further systematic threat to clinic ceremony came from
the presence in most settings of an audience to the interaction between parents, child and doctor. In my earlier
discussion of this audience, I emphasized the variety of
procedures that were used to minimize its effect upon the
consultation. Students or other staff were typically
placed to one side of the action, and conversation with
them was carefully controlled. Not only was the use of
the clinical format restricted but the version in which it
appeared was sober and sanitized. Nevertheless, despite
these various attempts to moderate its influence, the
presence of an audience routinely altered the nature of
consultations and undercut the idealized version of a
private, confidential and uniquely focussed relationship.
The presence of an audience gave the proceedings a very
public air. The settings were not made for the easy revelation of matters of great intimacy. Staff did not assume

a confidential manner, for it was plain that nothing was
in confidence;   anything that was said was available for
discussion, if not now then later on.   This lack of
privacy was most marked in the large wards of the maternity hospital.   As has been seen, the round had some of the
aspects of a show, but this was a show not just for the
individual mother and her child but for all the other
mothers present in the ward, who watched the round's
progress with some interest.   A discussion between the
doctor and one mother could set this other audience
talking loudly amongst themselves:

> Dr K: How do you manage to look so good?   You've got a
>   marvellous hairstyle.
> Mother: (blushing) Well ... fairly....
> Dr K: Have you done anyone else's hair while you've
>   been here?
> Mother: Oh, just one.
> 2nd Mother: She makes us all look like drudges.
> 3rd Mother: She must get up at 4 o'clock to do it.

Audiences did not normally talk amongst themselves or
comment on the action, but their mere presence transformed
the occasion.   Teaching in particular had a striking
force, regardless of whether any individual child was
actually taught on in the presence of its parents.   The
importance of teaching in many of these settings was
enshrined in their actual construction.   Outpatient
clinics were designed to accommodate particular types of
teaching, and as teaching styles varied so too did their
ecology.   The 'amphitheatre' was built to enable patients
to be treated as clinical material and had a stage,
floodlights and banked seats for that purpose.   Even where
teaching was less overtly the dominant activity, its
impact could still be reflected in the bricks and mortar
of the setting.   The suite of three rooms in the Scottish
hospital clinics and the cubicle system in the American
hospital both enabled teaching and clinical discussion to
form a regular part of outpatient work.   Even though they
might say nothing, the audience on these occasions could
be very large.   Six or seven students sat in on some of
the Scottish hospital clinics, while the numbers in the
amphitheatre clinic could reach as many as thirty.   On
entering these settings, parents were immediately presented with a mass of faces, all watching them with interest.   Indeed, in the amphitheatre they were quite literally on stage:

> (Father, mother and child enter floodlit stage.)
> Mother: (nervously) Hello.

    Dr W: (sitting in front row) This is your first child,
        isn't it?

    Dr W: And there weren't any other problems?
    Mother: No, she's fine otherwise. It really floored us
          when we walked in to see all these people here.
    Dr W: Uh-huh. OK. You can put her up on the couch.
        (Mother does so. Three doctors get up from their
        seats and go up on to the stage.)

Parents had normally no real choice as to the presence
of an audience. In many settings they were there for each
and every case. It is true that the objections made by
one mother after a consultation in the Scottish neurological clinic led to the doctor banning students from
that clinic, but this was the only mother whose criticism
was mentioned by staff and even she did not object during
the clinic itself. Since the hospital was a teaching
hospital there was no possibility of banning students from
more than one or two of the more specialist clinics. Although teaching while parents were present was typically
limited, doctors did not normally seek permission for this
except in the most serious cases.
There was in fact one setting, the maternity hospital
ward-round, where requests and apologies of a kind were
routinely made; but these were not phrased in such a
manner as to permit ready refusal, as witness these quotations from the beginning, middle and end of a consultation in which the doctor supervised the standard examination of a newborn baby:

    Dr K: Hello, Mrs Mackie. We've come to look at your
        baby. (To baby) Here's a big audience to look
        at you. (To mother) Do sit down, Mrs Mackie and
        you won't tire yourself. Don't worry, we'll move
        baby near you for the examination.

    Dr K: (to student) You just do it and we'll comment on
        what you've missed. You won't mind, will you,
        because it's the only way to learn. (To mother)
        And you won't mind either, will you, because
        we've all got to get experience.

After the student has finished the examination and Dr K
has commented on this:

    Dr K: (to mother) Your baby's super, Mrs Mackie. You
        don't mind putting up with all this, do you? And
        she's a very good little patient. (Mother smiles
        weakly, and looks exhausted.)

When teaching was done it took up an important part of
the time allocated to the patients. For example, of the
four special nursery follow-up clinics that were observed,
two contained students and two did not. Cases in the
latter clinics lasted between eight and ten minutes,
whereas those where students were present lasted no more
than five minutes. Where teaching was carried out in the
presence of the child even less time was allocated directly to parents. Some staff summarized the history of a
case after the parents had arrived and made occasional
comments to students during it. On some occasions where
parents were keen to stay and full of questions, doctors
still ended the case rapidly, in order to address the
students' questions instead.

The domination of the action by teaching was at its
most extreme in the maternity hospital ward-round.
Indeed, in some of these cases it would be more accurate
to talk of the mother, and not the students, as consti-
tuting the audience.

Teaching had other effects besides these. Even where
doctors never openly taught in front of patients and where
the segregation of teaching and treating was apparently
complete, the mere presence of a student audience could
transform each case into teaching material. The action
that apparently centred on the child and its parents had
a dual role; the doctors were not simply doing diagnosis
and treatment, they were also demonstrating how to do
these tasks. Such demonstration was done by first telling
students what to see in the interaction they were about to
witness, and then enacting it in such a way as to make the
lesson visible; a feat which enabled yet further teaching
to be done on the case once it had been processed.
Conversations that took place solely with parents might,
in consequence, be thoroughly informed by the requirements
of teaching. In some cases topics were inserted which
were of relevance only to the students.

For example, Dr F used the cases in the special nursery
follow-up clinic as a general resource to teach students
about normal babies. Each case was used to illustrate one
particular aspect of a normal baby, with the aim of
building up a composite picture by the end of the clinic.
Since there was no guarantee that the babies who turned
up would match each of the aspects to be considered, the
choice of a baby to illustrate any one feature was often
arbitrary. In the following instance the doctor had been
teaching about smiling prior to the baby's arrival. The
baby was already known to be smiling but nevertheless,
although the consultation lasted only four minutes, the
doctor used the opportunity (a) to show how to check on

'real' smiles;   (b) to reveal the normal age at which
babies smile;   (c) to show how to produce a social smile:

> Dr F: Now, the last time we saw him I think he was
>   smiling. Is he smiling? Really?
> Grandmother: Yes.
> Dr F: You're sure it's not wind?
> Grandmother: No.
>
> Dr F: He smiled at eight weeks, didn't he?
> Grandmother: Yes.
>
> Dr F: (to baby) Hello, hello. (Baby smiles. To
>   students) You get easy social smiles. (To baby)
>   Come on, give us a smile, give us a smile, give
>   us a smile.... (To grandmother) And he laughs
>   and chuckles, does he?
> Grandmother: Yes.

The imposition of such a rigid teaching format was
found only when the doctor faced a similar kind of task
in case after case, as in those settings where developmental assessment was routinely done. In other clinics
doctors taught from whatever happened to turn up, from
'inside' a case, although still relating this to what they
would normally expect to see. But however it was done the
impact of teaching was considerable. This was particularly true of the American hospital's ambulatory clinics.
The patients waiting in their cubicles were auxiliaries
to a floating classroom, for right in the centre of the
clinic the doctors, interns and residents had a private
room from which they worked, taught and learned. For
them, this was where the day's action centred and their
interaction with parents was informed by the manners
peculiar to that classroom:

> Mother: This kid has had everything done to her. (She
>   describes various tests and then mentions that
>   her teeth were slow to come through.)
> Dr O: Where did they do this?
> Mother: St Cyprian's.
> Dr O: Oh. (To resident) When the teeth are slow what's
>   the first thing you think of? (He smiles and
>   waits.) Just like that! (He snaps his fingers.
>   Resident does not answer.) Hypothyroidism!

In such instances there was an important sense in which
the parents, the child and the doctor were all on display
for the benefit of others, a sense which might undercut

the primary assumption that consultations were for the
child's benefit. More subtly perhaps, the physical
presence of such an audience could make it yet more
difficult still for parents to discuss their child and
its problems. To do so was hard enough, given their medical ignorance and their fear of seeming foolish, but such
uncertainties were only compounded by a setting in which
informed medical discussion was so patently an integral
part. In any consultation parents ran the risk of being
covertly judged, but where students or other staff were
present such judgment was clearly a central part of the
medical agenda, even if it was carried out in private.

Quite apart from the more subtle intrusions of the
audience, not all attempts to subordinate and segregate
this other action were in fact successful. Three particular difficulties may be noted: the technical problems of
managing the same interaction for different audiences;
the difficulties of physical segregation, and the problem
of controlling equals. Doctors in fact might have three
or even four separate audiences, each of whom had to be
taken into account in some way. Students required one
thing and mothers another, nurses might need instructions
and researchers needed information. To do all these
things simultaneously and to examine and treat the patient
as well was not easy. For beginners, conversing with
mothers might be difficult. One registrar who examined
children on the maternity hospital ward-round not only
took far longer to do the actual examination but also
complained afterwards, 'I just don't know how to talk to
mothers yet.' Even those who were practised in such situations might still omit to take all the members of their
differing audiences into account simultaneously. Here,
for instance, Dr F, in trying to combine both teaching and
consulting, uses a series of terms such as 'unusual',
'damage' and 'surprise' which were never normally said to
parents in such circumstances:

    Dr F: How old was he then?
    Mother: Five months ... (pause) ... Oh, they both had
           chicken-pox.
    Dr F: Really! That's very unusual.
    Mother: My oldest son brought it home from school. I
           had four of them with it at the same time and
           associated with it they had an irritating dry
           cough which he's had ever since.
    Dr F: Yes, chicken-pox can cause a bit of lung damage
           at the time. That's not a surprise. As you
           know, chicken-pox is normally mild.
    Mother: Yes.

Apart from these technical problems, physical segregation could sometimes be problematic. Even where clinics
were relatively private, as in the Scottish settings,
doors were sometimes left ajar, and in the maternity
hospital privacy was very hard to find. Mothers were to
be found in the corridors as well as in the beds, and Dr K
urged the students to caution, reminding them that 'even
the walls have ears in the Matty'. The American clinics
faced the greatest problems here. The cubicles in which
parents sat were windowless and too small for the door to
remain shut for long, while the room from which staff
worked had no door at all. In consequence some consultations took place with the door open, while the supposedly private talk of staff in the corridor and operations
room could sometimes be overheard in the cubicles.
Finally, it should be noted that not all doctors
actually wished to subordinate all other action to that
with the parents, while in some instances other staff
would not let them. On several occasions when staff of
some equivalence to the doctor sat in on a clinic they
assumed rights to intervene and discuss that were never
granted to students or nurses. More generally, in the
American amphitheatre clinics and in one of the Scottish
hospital clinics, patient and parents, though still
perhaps primus inter pares constituted only a part of the
agenda under consideration. (3) Other staff and nurses
might discuss things among themselves, if quietly, and,
in line with this greater prominence of the clinical
format, the atmosphere in the clinic was both technical
and informal; jokes were made, journals cited and gossip
exchanged. This point should not be over-emphasized. The
backstage medicine that was revealed was still a selective
version of the medical world. Nevertheless, it was
different from that which was normally revealed, as
witness the following quotation from a Scottish clinic.
In this consultation the doctor had spent ten minutes
talking to parents about their child's retardation, explaining that he felt it most unlikely that their child
would attend a normal school. All of a sudden he noticed
a registrar hovering in the background:

Dr H: (to registrar) Sorry, you've been waiting while
      I've been chattering. (Registrar hands Dr H an
      X-ray.) It's still a bit spotty; could they
      come back in six weeks' time, it could mean
      cystic fibrosis. Sorry, I didn't see you coming
      in. Have you been there long? I am sorry, help
      yourself to another patient because this really
      requires a bit of explanation.

MEDICAL INCAPACITY

In considering the divorce between the rhetoric of the
bureaucratic format and what was in fact on offer, some
attention must be paid to medical incapacity. Unlike the
tensions discussed so far, this was not a universal difficulty, for many medical problems were solved. Nevertheless, some conditions were difficult to cure or amelio-
rate, and in others there was no cure at all. Some of
the special difficulties that this failure created have
already been discussed, but a more general point remains
to be considered. I have noted the way in which our
culture divides the world into natural and social spheres.
On this analysis medical incapacity, so long as it is not
simply a matter of personal incompetence, and so long as
there are no other more viable methods, cannot strictly
be judged in moral terms. Medicine may have failed but
it is more a case of Nature defeating Man than of personal
or professional dereliction. Children are not artificial
products for whom we can hold the manufacturers or the
mechanics responsible when they go wrong.
     Nevertheless, there are senses in which it seems le-
gitimate to talk of moral failure, even when there is no
question of a merely personal inadequacy. Take, for
example, the following comment, which followed a consultation in which a mother had denounced the medical service
and praised the Doman-Delcato method:

> Dr I: As she says, we stand indicted. We haven't been
>   able to do anything for her here. We just see
>   her every three months and say, 'How are things?'
>   'Oh, much the same,' she says. And I say,
>   'Right, I'll see you next time.'

Similarly Dr I confessed to another mother, as he broke
the news of her child's severe retardation, 'I feel such a
fraud.' To feel fraudulent or stand indicted is to accept
the validity of moral judgment in these cases, and such
opinion seems related to a basic belief about science
which permeates our culture. In this, the constraints of
the natural sphere are acknowledged but it is also held
that, through the application of human thought and experiment, the natural will become known and socialized. On
this analysis, all phenomena both should and will become
subject to human intervention and modification. Scientific medicine has been amongst the most striking examples
of this plan of investigation and alteration, and its
sales pitch is based upon its increasing ability to intervene within the natural on its customers' behalf. Where

striking advances had been made both doctor and parent
could rejoice in its success:

> Dr F: (to researcher) This baby was very ill at birth.
>   She was nine weeks early and had very severe
>   hyaline membrane infection. We had to put her
>   on the ventilator. She was pretty ill in every
>   respect. Now she's fine in every respect.
>   (Grinning at baby) You're lucky you weren't born
>   twenty years earlier, my girl.
> Mother: (laughing) Otherwise, you'd be dead.
>
> Dr F: (as mother gets up to leave) A triumph of modern
>   medicine.

Given these human hopes in the progress and capacity of
medicine, problems for which there were no solutions could
undermine its credibility. All that parents could be
offered was that 'one day' medicine might have the answer,
but such consolation was of little use to parents whose
children had such problems now. (4) This failure to meet
the implicit claims of high-technology medicine resulted
in, or was compounded by, a series of other features, all
of which might reinforce a sense of defeat and thus
threaten the overall meaning of the consultation. If
established medicine had no ready answers this left the
field open to its competitors, to parental pressure groups
such as that for autism or to non-establishment medicine
like the Doman-Delcato method. Just as parents might feel
cheated when medicine could do little, so staff could find
working with such cases an equally depressing experience.
It was pleasant to administer triumphs, less so to admit
failure. Here in a quotation from fieldnotes a doctor
is talking enthusiastically about success:

> Dr McIntosh said that he had worked 32 hours that
> weekend but it was worth it because he liked to see the
> results. He'd had two meningitis cases and had also
> been involved in saving a baby's life. He had worked
> out what was wrong when it came into casualty and had
> managed to get treatment underway immediately. Areas
> of medicine where you couldn't get good results, for
> example, geriatrics, handicap and psychiatry, didn't
> interest him very much.

Thus in chronic conditions such as handicap the criteria of success had to be totally altered from those that
prevailed elsewhere. Others have noted how parents alter
their time-scale and look for small rewards (Voysey,

1975). A similar process was essential for medical staff
if they were to gain any satisfaction from handling such
cases:

> Dr J: There's a tendency to think of chronic handicap
> as the least interesting aspect (of paediatrics)
> because the rewards are so small and because
> there's a general feeling that you can't do much
> anyway.... I like to feel that I'm achieving
> something and it's less easy to feel that in this
> sort of clinic. What I have learnt is that, if
> you look for small gains, and that if your
> expectations are realistic, small gains can be
> as rewarding as major cures in general paedi-
> atrics.

Such redefinition might prove difficult, as might the
other strategy in which staff engaged, that of switching
from a therapeutic to a managerial role. The rationale
here was that, even if cures could not be provided, at
least some other form of help might be given. But although paediatricians might broaden their remit, they
lacked control over non-medical resources. They themselves were not responsible for assessing whether a child
should go to a normal school, nor had they any real say
over access to nursery places, to special schools or to
special institutional care. They had no authority to
provide special housing or to find money for special
clothes, furniture or toys. Yet such matters might be of
far more practical importance than the little that they
themselves could offer. Doctors might take it upon themselves to inquire about all these wider things and to
contact the relevant authorities, but they were distant
from the real sources of power.
Even the limited things that medicine itself had to
offer could still place extreme burdens on some parents.
Certain chronic medical conditions demanded continual
parental care, special therapy by parents, and regular
attendance at several different outpatient clinics; very
often for no great reward. As such, medical services
might be both overwhelming and fundamentally disappoint-
ing, as one doctor remarked when discussing severe cerebral palsy:

> Dr I: Orthodox medicine hasn't got very much to offer
> apart from physiotherapy to those parents who
> want something to do. In fact, there's a greater
> variety of parents of handicapped children than
> there is of handicap. Large numbers of parents

won't do anything, they won't even bring the
child up to the hospital. Either they can't get
it organized or they're just not able to do this.
Very often it's a single-parent family or if it
is two parents they're both at work and it's just
too difficult to arrange. For them orthodox
medicine provides almost too much, and yet for
Mrs Miller it doesn't provide enough.... Now
she's doing so much that she's almost harming
herself. She's searching for more and more to
do, and a lot of medicine is just palliative.

Finally, in considering the strains that medical incapacity posed for the ceremonial order of the clinic, some
mention should be made of those problems to which there
were certainly technical solutions but which could present
major practical difficulties in their implementation.
Several of these have already been discussed. There were,
for example, the unwillingness to investigate parental
theories of aetiology, and the discrepancy between the
implicit assumption of a more personal relationship and
the anonymity of medical work in large bureaucracies. And
things might not even get this far. The very offer of
help might well be rejected by parents, since to accept it
was to define their child as handicapped.
To these difficulties one more should be added. I have
already discussed the complex way in which bad news was
broken. Looked at from another angle this could also be
seen, not as a search for agreement as I described it
earlier, but as a lack of frankness. For doctors displayed no such qualms in less serious cases. In his
intensive study of 14 children with poliomyelitis, Davis
(1963) argued that, in the less severe cases, medical
staff revealed far more at a much earlier date. This
finding was confirmed across the whole range of cases and
clinics in this present study. Just as doctors used
dramatic language only for trivial complaints such as
septic spots, so too they were immediately frank about the
less severe problems which they encountered. Here for
instance a doctor discusses a urinary infection that he
has just diagnosed:

Dr G: Now these urinary infections in little girls are
quite difficult to get rid of. There's nothing
serious usually but it's worth while checking up
that there's nothing wrong with her kidneys, and
that means doing an X-ray and we'll also get a
sample of urine sent off to see if it's infected.
The best thing is to arrange for her to have an

X-ray and I'll see you again in a month's time.
If something is wrong then we need to do
something about it. If there's not anything
wrong then we'll still need her to attend to see
what's going on. I might have to see her
repeatedly. The treatment might take as long as
six months. I'm afraid there's no easy way
around this. We need to stop it now. There's
no easy answer provided by clinical medicine but
it's best to do it now so that it stops re-
curring.

Similarly, here is how a doctor broke the news in a
case of relatively mild cerebral palsy. Again this was
the child's first visit to the hospital and, unlike the
more serious cases considered earlier, the future was
spelt out very directly:

Dr I: She does walk but her walking is never going to
be, um, well, perfect. She'll always be adequate
on her feet but I don't think she'll ever be able
to walk long distances.
(Mother looks upset and goes very red.)

Despite this crucial difference in the extent to which
doctors revealed information, it should be noted that even
in the less serious cases staff were not completely open
with parents. Not only did they conceal the inner
workings of medicine but, since the future was always
unclear and many conditions were no more than remote statistical possibilities, they routinely suppressed any
marginal doubts that they might have about a child.
Indeed, this bowdlerization was practised even where staff
were legally obliged to be frank. The consultants in the
Scottish hospital were required to assess all children
being considered for adoption and to produce a detailed
medical report for the benefit of the social work department, the magistrates and the prospective parents.
Yet here too they concealed certain doubts where they felt
it to be necessary:

Dr G: (speaking to the adopting mother and social
worker, after filling out a form for the magistrates) ... I certainly think everything's all
right.... I can't find any abnormalities so
it'll be through by the end of January.

Dr G: (afterwards) ... That was a difficult one. I'd
have been happier if she'd reacted to the rattle

> and happier if she'd lifted her head up earlier.
> She did it in the end but I felt she could have
> done it earlier.   One has also got to take into
> account that she is an Indian baby, they might
> be slower to develop.   Negroes, of course, are
> faster.   One has also got to take into account
> the reason why she's adopting this baby.   She
> may be one of those people who have a thing about
> underprivileged children.   I would like to see
> her again in two or three months' time perhaps
> but, as she seems to be so set on this thing, I
> won't implant the doubt in her mind.   But she
> seemed a pretty lively thing.

This general difficulty in being frank constituted the
last of those tensions which systematically informed any
and every medical consultation.   However trivial the
condition there was always the possibility that the doctor
was not being completely open in what he or she said about
it, a possibility that was strengthened by the brevity
with which these matters were normally considered.   Such
strain was kept well below the surface on most occasions,
and was only visible in the more serious cases where
parents too found their doubts hard to discuss and the
relevant questions difficult to put.   'Will she ever grow
out of it?'   'Will he catch up?'   'Will she ever walk?' -
all these were usually asked in a manner quite different
from other kinds of inquiry.   They were said with embarrassment or with defiance, mumbled or barked and
generally treated as awkward, both for themselves and for
doctors.

EASY ALLIANCES

In considering the sources of ease and tension within the
bureaucratic format, I began with the latter since these
were systematic features of any medical consultation.
There was, in other words, the permanent possibility of
a serious disjunction between the ceremony and the
substance of such occasions.   Staff were constrained both
to investigate their clients' competence and morality and
to preserve their good name.   Likewise, parents were
obliged both to reveal their doubts and problems and to
ensure that they did not waste staff's time or challenge
their authority.
   In consequence, for the alliance to be of any ease,
somewhat special conditions were required.   The fewest
difficulties occurred where there was no medical problem

and no expectation of one on either side. Routine developmental screening in the local authority and city clinics was typically a pleasant, humorous affair where mothers and doctors joined in mutual admiration of the young child (Davis and Strong, 1976b). Overtly, the medical interaction served as merely an occasion for such activity. Wonderment and joy were legitimately displayed even prior to medical inspection, and tests were simply tricks which enabled a child to display its virtuosity.

In more standard forms of consultation where there was a medical problem of some kind, it obviously helped if the condition was trivial or easily cured. Moreover, the less reliance that staff needed to place upon the parents, either for information or for care, then the easier their relationship could become. There was one important exception to this rule for, in the right circumstances, medical dependence upon parents might lead to an extremely close alliance. Such conditions were found in some cases involving drug therapy and in some of the milder cases treated by the occupational and physiotherapy departments. Here parents might be given an important but relatively simple part to play, something which was their own and which depended on their motivation and skill but which stood a good chance of success. In such cases, it was common for staff not merely to treat parents as allies but to formulate them as such. Here is an example from a Scottish general medical clinic where the child is suffering from encopresis:

> Dr H: So we're well on the way to winning but we've not found the right adjustment yet.
> Mother: As I say, I've been giving him 20ml a day but that turned out to be too much.
> Dr H: Too much?
> Mother: Yes, it was like dirty water. We gave it a try but it wasn't any good....
> Dr H: Well, I feel we've reached the stage where you're almost the doctor and I'm just watching what you're doing.

And here is another from physiotherapy:

> Therapist A: Well, I think the reason she's come on so far by herself is just due to you doing this sort of thing with her. I think that's what's done it. That's what's brought her on this far.
> Mother: Well, I've learnt a lot already.

In replying in this modest fashion the mother paid due deference to the alliance and recognized her subordinate relationship within it. Here then was a nice allocation of praise by both parties. In more serious cases where doctors could do little, an easy alliance depended on parents' open acceptance both of the facts of the case and of medical limitations. Even the most 'sensible' parents took time to adjust. When they did so alliances of some ease could on occasion be managed; doctors might compliment a child without any danger of such praise being taken as a warrant of the child's normality, and parents might criticize the service without staff taking this as any personal challenge. (5)

It must be emphasized that many apparently easy relationships rested on a distinctly shaky base. Their surface smoothness and even celebration was premised on the avoidance of some important matters and parental ignorance as to others. Here for example is a brief description of a close alliance during one consultation with Dr I. The patient was a nine-year-old girl with epilepsy:

1 When the parents arrived in the clinic the doctor asked the mother if she would mind summarizing her daughter's medical history for the benefit of the students present, a task that doctors normally reserved for themselves.

2 Later the mother introduced the topic of a book on epilepsy that the doctor had recommended. She talked about this enthusiastically and the doctor joined her in this, adding his own comments.

3 Unlike most mothers, this one let her daughter speak at length in answer to the doctor's questions and, when she herself discussed her child with the doctor, she continually looked towards her daughter to check the accuracy of her remarks.

4 After hearing how the child had fared since her last visit, the doctor presented future management as something to be jointly decided upon - 'I'm not sure but I feel inclined to let it go for a bit' (i.e. to continue without medication) - 'How do you feel about this?'

Epilepsy was a condition in whose management parents had a major role to play. They monitored the child's progress and were responsible for seeing that drugs were taken daily. There were, however, additional unspoken grounds for the alliance to be so strongly expressed here. The girl had been very seriously ill after a previous drug treatment and the doctor had every incentive to share re-

sponsibility for managing the condition with the parents.
Further, although the mother did most of the talking, her
husband was also present. He only came occasionally but
it was he who always asked the awkward questions, in this
case 'Will she ever grow out of it?' Such a division of
labour enabled the wife to play the part of loyal ally and
safeguarded her future relations with the doctor. No
detailed reply was actually given to the father's
question. The doctors suspected that the attacks might
turn out to be temporal lobe epilepsy and possibly permanent, but there was no clear way of knowing until the
child reached adolescence. Thus, as Dr J commented after
a visit from them nearly two years later:

> Dr J: They're not worrying nearly enough about the
> future ... but you can't really tell them off
> otherwise they won't tell you the truth and it's
> very, very important to get at the truth. It's
> very difficult to know how to play such cases.

The nurse entered the room and said she had just heard the
parents telling the girl how nice the doctor was.

PROFESSIONAL MOTHERS

In summary, although there were circumstances in which
alliances could be made with some ease the possibility of
tension was always there. In fact the only sorts of
mothers with whom staff routinely had an easy alliance,
almost regardless of the circumstances of the case, were
not natural mothers at all but foster-mothers. Foster-
mothers were the ideal client precisely because they were
not parents, but colleagues and junior colleagues at that.
    In all, 17 foster-mothers were observed in a total of
26 consultations. (6) Those patients who were in the care
of these foster-mothers were mostly babies, and only six
children were seen, their ages ranging from between two
and eight. Most fostered babies were quickly adopted and,
whatever the reason for their attendance, their fitness
for adoption was a central theme in most settings, even
if this was not always openly discussed.
    When compared with natural mothers, foster-mothers had
several distinct advantages as medical allies. Whereas
parents were only supposed to be competent and caring,
these qualities could normally be assumed in foster-
mothers. Indeed they were essential qualifications for
the job and as such implicitly guaranteed by their em-
ployers. This is not to say that doctors placed immediate

trust in foster-mothers, and it was common for them to begin by checking the number of children that the mother had fostered. But once a certain level of experience had been established all could proceed with relative ease, for immediate weight could be given to what they said. Here is an excerpt from the beginning of a case in the neurological clinic:

> Dr J: You have children of your own?
> Foster-mother: Yes, one, and I've had nine foster-children.
> Dr J: Ah, well, your opinion is worth its weight in gold.

Similarly a foster-mother's visit to a clinic where students were present was often an occasion for stressing that one must pay careful attention to what they said:

> Dr G: ... I thought he was a little slow. His head was falling back a little early. I asked the foster-mother - they must be very experienced women who've had a lot of babies, one gets very acute answers from them - I asked her what she thought. He was a little slower than others she'd had, which is a very significant thing. So the adoption was postponed.

Doctors relied on foster-mothers in this way, not just because they were experienced but also because they were emotionally detached. Indeed, for the job to stay a job they had to remain so. As one foster-mother said at the end of a session:

> I hope it's quick (the adoption). I told the social worker that I wanted it to be as quick as possible, as I'm getting far too attached to her. I hope it's done within a month.

Because of their normal emotional distance, foster-mothers could discuss their charges in quite distinctive ways. On the one hand their lack of long-term commitment to the children meant that they could display a very open affection towards them, or at least towards the babies, all of whom received far more overt affection than was normally given by natural mothers. With natural mothers, such display could be read as evidence of an overwhelming attachment which might render technical discussion of the child's condition problematic; but not with foster-mothers. On the contrary, doctors felt able to use a

clinical format in their presence, treating them as they
did their other professional colleagues. Where they had
worries about a child, both doctor and foster-mother could
speak about them freely and in very similar terms. Thus
great affection could be readily combined with a much
greater emotional distance than was usual. Medical
problems were not potential tragedies for either party,
merely unfortunate things about which one might be worried
or even upset, but only in a professional kind of way.
Doctors' incapacity in some cases was of no great personal
consequence and, since the child was not the foster-
mother's ultimate responsibility, a serious condition
threatened no major blight upon her life. Since she was
not the child's actual mother she could not normally blame
herself for its condition.

In such circumstances the impersonal bureaucratic
setting of the consultations was a source of far less
tension. The infrequency of visits to hospital clinics,
the brief time available for each to be accomplished, the
gap in formal education and social class that was often
present, the formal agenda and formal surroundings and
the obtrusive nature of official records and recording:
each of these features could increase the distance between
doctor and parent. Yet with foster-mothers such bureaucratic arrangements were a part of and might even enhance
their status. The foster-mother was a professional
herself and her responsibility towards the child was
arranged on a bureaucratic basis. To be treated in a
formal manner was simply part of the job. Since doctors
commonly treated them with great respect and often deferred to their experience and expertise, their visits to
the clinic could be a professionally rewarding experience.
(7) Bureaucratic arrangements were best suited to those
who were themselves at least partly bureaucrats.

At the same time, although foster-mothers were in a
sense the doctor's colleagues they did not represent the
independent and competitive threat to medical authority
that was typical of some discussion in the clinical
format. Their knowledge, though extensive, was derived
from experience rather than professional training and as
such they were clearly subordinate to medical staff. On
no occasion did a foster-mother challenge a doctor and,
although some emphasized their individual agreement with
doctors' observations, none placed any stress on the
distinctive quality of their own judgment or claimed any
special rights in their children.

Their behaviour therefore contrasts strongly both with
that of natural mothers and with that of some other professionals who accompanied children on occasion. This

latter group of social workers and house-mothers shared
the foster-mothers' professional detachment but most of
them lacked their detailed knowledge of the particular
child, while, as was seen in the case of the social worker
who accompanied the mentally retarded mother, some of them
posed a distinct threat to the doctor's own authority.
Social workers did not define themselves as subordinates
but as equals and claimed their own special competences
and rights in the child, claims that were not made by
foster-mothers. (8) Given the subordinate but insider
status of the latter, doctors could relax more freely with
them. Indeed, whereas no doctor ever criticized another
doctor to a natural mother or to a social workers, one
general practitioner received heavy criticism when the
child was represented by a foster-mother.

Given these features, and the additional fact that
foster-mothers were a scarce and valuable resource and
thus to be encouraged, such consultations were not only
easy affairs but they took on a different form from those
found with natural mothers. As competent but junior professionals, foster-mothers did not so much raise problems
with doctors as make semi-formal reports on their observations. Consultations were typically straight to the
point. Doctors asked immediately what they had observed
and foster-mothers replied in a careful and detached
manner. Several of these points, the status of foster-
mothers' evidence, the manner in which they reported
rather than simply spoke, and their considerable emotional
detachment are revealed in the following two quotations
from the beginning and end of a consultation. Here we may
see a clinical rather than a bureaucratic format:

    Dr G: Hello.
    FM/SW: Hello.
    Dr G: Now, how long have you been fostering him for?
    FM: Yes, six weeks.
    Dr G: Since a few days after he was born, isn't it?
    FM: Yes. I noticed he was a bit slow.
    Dr G: In what way?
    FM: Well, he was a bit wobbly, a bit slow to smile and
        his balance is bad.
    Dr G: And is he smiling now?
    FM: Yes.
    Dr G: Of course, it is normal to be wobbly at this age.
    FM: Yes, it is.

    Dr G: Well, there are just one or two things. There's
        an annoying little heart murmur. There's also
        his posture; he was a little bit floppy when I
        held him up.

SW: Yes.
Dr G: I'd be a little uneasy about that, but then
      someone has to be below average, and what do you
      do about it?
SW: Well, we'll let Mrs Miller (foster-mother) keep him
    (for the time being).
FM: Yes, I'd like to keep him.   I'm not happy about it.
Dr G: No, I'm not either.

The relative ease with which consultations with foster-
mothers were conducted emphasizes yet again the many
tensions that underlay paediatric consultations with
parents. Of course not every consultation was a tense
occasion and some clinics were relaxed, even jolly, affairs. But, as we have seen, doctor-parent interaction
was often a most complex matter. Discussion was circuitous and guarded, words had to be carefully chosen,
messages must be indirect. Even the easy alliances had
to be made with care and, although one might still stand
on ceremony, the somewhat rickety structure beneath one's
feet did shake alarmingly from time to time.

8 Conclusions and generalizations

A fairly standard and not unreasonable response to a
detailed sociological description of some small segment
of the world is 'so what?' Description can become an end
in itself and, in so far as there is any pleasure in the
rigours of analysis and writing, most of the joy comes
from making one small piece fit with another and tidying
up all the loose ends. (In this respect ethnography has
a good deal in common with housework.) These obsessions
are rarely shared by readers, who are more concerned with
the point of the whole enterprise. And here the analyst
is faced with a problem, for the conclusions,which may be
drawn from a description such as this are at many different levels, while the evidence for much of what one wants
to say is strictly limited, case studies not lending
themselves too well to the sociological urge to explain
the world in a swift paragraph.

This final chapter has therefore a rather jumbled and
somewhat tentative character, for in it I shall essay a
considerable variety of rather difficult tasks: a recon-
sideration of Goffman's work on frames; a suggestion as
to the extent to which the bureaucratic format is in
general medical use; a hypothesis as to its origins;
and finally some discussion of its possible drawbacks.
Here then is a wide range of topics about which I can only
offer suggestions rather than draw definite conclusions.
Nevertheless, to make the whole thing readable I shall
often abandon caution, in so far as this is compatible
with a modicum of academic respectability.

I shall begin with some comments on Goffman, though
once again the non-sociologist may prefer to pass rapidly
on to the next section.

FRAME ANALYSIS

In introducing the concept of role format I spent a little time in considering Goffman's own approach to the analysis of interaction. Having analysed one particular role format in some detail, as well as reflecting on some of its rivals, we may now go back to Goffman's work and see if we have learnt any general lessons about frame analysis.

Before we do this it may be useful to summarize Goffman's interests in this area. The first point to note is that although Goffman's approach to interaction is fundamentally structural he has in fact devoted relatively little attention to the analysis of particular frames. While Gonos (1977) is therefore right in describing frames as the basis of Goffman's vision, and indeed his analysis is a valuable corrective to many previous interpretations, his article is misleading if it is taken as a guide to what Goffman actually does.

To write such a guide is a most tricky enterprise but, in essence, Goffman's interest in frames themselves has been restricted to the following four areas: first, to the general procedures by which *any* frame is established; (1) second, to the ways in which a frame may serve as an original against which copies or transformations of various kinds can be made, such as jokes, dreams, deceptions, experiments, rehearsals, demonstrations and plays (Goffman, 1975a); third, to an emphasis that frames represent a moral as well as a cognitive order; and finally, to the delineation of certain very broad classes of frame, like those distinctions between natural and social frames, focussed and unfocussed interaction that were considered in chapter 1.

This is in itself a formidable body of work. However, it must be noted that Goffman's method for studying frames is quite different from the one that I have used here. His work is largely of the essay form, and is typically based, not on the detailed observation and recording of particular frames, but on the consideration of a huge variety of different frames studied through close attention to the materials of his daily life and through very wide reading. Conventional fieldwork has played a part in all this but only a part, for one of Goffman's basic aims has been to produce a series of very basic propositions which relate to all frames, universal generalizations which hold true regardless of time and place; and for this project what is most needed are first, a wide range of comparative materials and second, illustrations which have an unusually dramatic power - frames which have the capacity to illuminate the workings of all others.

It is this latter concern which explains why games and
the theatre are the only two areas where Goffman has
studied particular frames in any detail, for these serve
as 'natural metaphors' (Garfinkel, 1956a) to reveal the
way in which all activities are framed. Their very arti-
ficiality, the fact that they are consciously framed in a
way in which other activities are not, can help us to
grasp the framing of more conventional matters.

The scope of Goffman's vision and his powerful use of
metaphor have added greatly to sociology. However, it
must be noted that, since the only distinctions he makes
between frames are at very high levels of abstraction, he
has nothing to say about many of the particular frames in
which sociologists and others have major substantive
interests. This is not to deny the great value of
Goffman's classifications, merely to observe that his
concerns, as he himself notes, are somewhat special.
Moreover, Goffman has another set of interests which are
in many ways as important as, or more important than his
concern with the frames themselves and which explain the
peculiar elusiveness of his work, touching on frames at
one moment only to dart away the next.

For Goffman, perhaps, the principal interest in frames
lies, not in their particular contents, nor in their
origins, nor indeed in their specific links with the wider
world of which they are a part, but in the relationship of
persons to frames. This concern is well stated in the
introduction to 'Interaction Ritual' (1972), though here
he picks out only one aspect of his interest in individuals and reality-construction:

> I assume that the proper study of interaction is not
> the individual and his psychology, but rather the syn-
> tactical relations among the acts of different persons
> mutually present to one another. Nonetheless since it
> is individual actors who contribute the ultimate
> material, it will always be reasonable to ask what
> general properties they must have if this sort of
> contribution is to be expected of them. What minimal
> model of the actor is needed if we are to wind him up,
> stick him in amongst his fellows and have an orderly
> type of traffic emerge.... Not then men and their
> moments. Rather moments and their men (Goffman, 1972,
> pp.2-3).

Two things should be noted about this statement, apart
that is from its elegant phrasing. First, that what
Goffman defines as the proper area of study for the
student of interaction, 'the syntactical relations among

the acts of different persons mutually present to one
another', is not in fact a field which he himself has
entered, save in passing, for to do so requires an interest in particular acts, identities and frames.

The second point is that this quotation highlights only
one aspect of Goffman's interest in individuals. In the
version presented here, people are mere creatures of
frames, and what we normally conceive of as a person is
reduced to a set of devices for the re-creation and
careful maintenance of pre-existing and super-ordinate
frames. (2) At the same time as offering us this
insightful but highly alienated vision of ourselves,
Goffman provides us with a quite separate model; one that
emphasizes the margins of freedom that allow the individual some space for his or her own interests, identity and
purposes.

Rather than being mere puppets, individuals, on this
other version, are shown to manipulate frames to their own
advantage (Goffman, 1971a), to make elaborate copies and
parodies of more serious frames (1975a), and to distance
themselves from frames even while acting within them. (3)
Indeed there is a strong moral emphasis in much of
Goffman's work and an anger at the way in which certain
disadvantaged individuals are treated as if they were no
more than the frame, or identity inside that frame, within
which others have encapsulated them (Goffman, 1968a,
1968b).

If these are Goffman's principal interests, much of the
task of frame analysis still remains to be done, though it
must be emphasized that what remains is in many ways the
easier and more conventional work. Despite this,
something may be gained from it, and in the next few pages
I shall attempt both some amendments and some additions
to the general model and suggest some propositions about
particular kinds of frame.

My first point concerns the extent to which individuals
are trapped within particular frames. As we have seen,
Goffman has gone to great lengths to establish the various
subtle ways in which people detach themselves from frames
and use them to their own purposes. This argument is
clearly supported by the data presented here. Parents who
disagreed with doctors would subtly alter their demeanour.
Similarly, despite the overt ban on moral investigation,
doctors could nevertheless still carry out complex reconstitutive work. At the same time we have also seen
that the extent and manner in which they could do this
were severely constrained. Goffman is aware that such
constraints exist but his very concern to establish that
there is a margin of freedom here may well mislead. There

is perhaps in his work an over-emphasis on the more
playful and free side of interaction. Certainly studies
such as 'Asylums' (1968a) and 'Stigma' (1968b) cannot be
viewed in this light, but these treat of special situations and identities, whereas in the more general discussions of the relationships of persons to frames there
is a tendency to see distance as always available, parody
and joking as a constant resource.

A good example of this tendency can be found in his
study of surgical team work (Goffman, 1961). (4) Here
Goffman explicitly treats the activity as a test-case, as
a situation in which above all we would expect to find a
total commitment to the role and thus a complete identifi-
cation with and control by the frame:

> Here, if anywhere in our society, we should find per-
> formances flushed with a feeling of the weight and
> dignity of their action. A Hollywood ideal is involved
> .... If the role perspective works, then, surely it
> works here, for in our society the surgeon, if anyone,
> is allowed and obliged to put himself into his work and
> get a self out of it (Goffman, 1961, p.116).

What in fact Goffman found there was a good deal of joking
and by-play; surgery was often conducted in a far from
serious manner. But to conclude from this that such major
role distance is a standard feature of frames is surely
mistaken, for there is no good reason to see this as a
test-case; indeed one might argue, following Goffman's
own work elsewhere (1971a), that it is precisely in a
back-stage area such as surgery that one would expect to
find large amounts of fun. The frame used in surgery is
another instance of the clinical format, a format which in
this study was often characterized by a high degree of
joking and distance, at least where it was used away from
patients. (One good example of this is the American case
conference which I cited at some length earlier on.)

By contrast, the bureaucratic format was a highly
serious affair. This is not to say that no joking ever
occurred - certain matters were indeed routinely laughed
about, for children were agreed to be an endless source of
amusement. But more fundamental things were treated with
considerable gravity. The doctor's competence and
authority were no laughing matter, nor indeed was the
child's illness. Only one mother tried to laugh off inquiries about her child's condition and make fun of the
doctor's remarks, and she was quickly humiliated by the
simple, serious repetition of the questions. It was
certainly possible to parody the frame on occasion or to

distance oneself from it, but the matters at stake were
too serious to allow for much leeway. Parents might show
a little non-verbal dissent but no more. The mother who
refused to play the ideal character ascribed to her was
investigated by social workers. Similarly, a doctor might
lightly parody his trade - 'a miracle of modern medicine'
- but only when an apparent miracle had in fact occurred.
Outside this context such a remark might constitute a
serious breach of frame, a sign that the doctor's attitude
was not all it might be.

In other words, although some distance was permitted on
occasion there were clear and important limits. Goffman
(1976b) has emphasized the 'dance' of interaction, the
movement to and from the frame; it is equally important
to note that there are usually clear rules on both the
amount and type of dancing and that there are many circumstances in which no more than a brief and stately minuet
is permitted. Moreover, even though he takes care to
emphasize the way in which role distance may in fact serve
the ultimate end of the activity system (1961), Goffman
still tends to write as if playing with frames or formats
was somehow separate from the frames, whereas I would see
such acts as governed by rules that are themselves part of
the form. Each format then contains within it guides for
respectable transformations and transgressions.

My second point concerns what Goffman has termed the
'syntactical relations' among the acts of individuals in
encounters. As I have argued, since he has not studied
the grammar of particular relationships he has left the
area almost untouched. Clearly a large number of case-
studies of different relationships would be required
before one could map out these things with any accuracy.
However, even with one study such as this, it does seem
possible to make a start on compiling a list of what the
basic elements in such a syntax would look like. (For a
related attempt at systematization, though in a slightly
different aream see Lofland, 1976.) That is, it seems
likely that there are a restricted number of components
out of which all role formats are constructed. I cannot
make any claims to comprehensiveness, but the following
six seemed crucial in the formats I have considered. Each
could vary independently of the others, and their particular combinations underlay the special nature of both individual formats and particular encounters.

1 The right to criticize: this may be allocated to
one, some, all or none of the participants. In the
bureaucratic and private formats it was the right of the
parents; in the charity format this prerogative belonged
to the doctor.

2 Where criticism is allowed, is character-work permitted and if so of what type, ameliorative or reconstitutive? (Reconstitutive character-work seems to carry a
much greater risk of challenges to the frame and is
therefore normally restricted to particular identities and
to highly formalized settings - at least as between
strangers.)

3 Who, if anyone, has rights to the overall control of
the interaction? (The central dimensions of power here
seem, at least in this study, to be: the range of legitimate objects of involvement for each participant; who
controls the setting, if anyone; who controls the timing,
sequencing and agenda, if anyone; who chooses the frame,
if anyone; within any one frame, who has rights to choose
identities both for themselves and for others; who can
authoritatively formulate what is going on; who controls
the criteria for admission to membership within the frame;
who can modify which rules.)

4 How far are topics, speaking-rights, etc. pre-
allocated? (For instance, it was normally doctors who
asked the questions and parents who did the answering, but
such rights are not an automatic indicator of control, for
on some occasions doctors asked parents to come along next
time with any questions they might have. In these latter
instances parents were pre-allocated the right to question
but overall control of the frame still lay with the
doctors.)

5 Are the participants of overtly equal competence in
the matter at hand or not?

6 What are the criteria which specify the qualifications necessary to be granted membership status within
the frame? (For example, although some situated roles
within formats are supposedly for anyone, that is anyone
can be a patient or client, not everyone in fact has the
particular competences or qualifications required.
Examples in this study were the Puerto Ricans who could
not speak English, the brother who accompanied a child
and, most importantly, child patients in general; none
of these quite fitted the demands of the bureaucratic
format as used here, and various other kinds of accommodation had to be devised.)

My third point also relates to the syntax of particular
kinds of frame, but in a somewhat different fashion. One
of Goffman's major concerns has been to specify the procedures and skills by which frames are maintained. But
since he has been interested only in propositions which
are universally true his approach is necessarily limited.
In this study the rule of irrelevance, that is the tacit
agreement to avoid all those things which might subvert

the reality of a particular frame, was indeed the basic
procedure by which formats were kept intact. Nevertheless, there were other methods of almost equal importance
which could not be understood without reference to the
syntax of particular formats. As we have seen, not everything that threatens a format can be avoided; the very
work of an activity system may run directly counter to its
ceremonial order, while that order itself may contain
contradictions: the rights, duties and character of one
status may conflict with those of another. Where such
contradictions occur, then means must be found for their
reconciliation if the activity system is to proceed
smoothly; and such means will themselves form an integral
part of the frame.

Once again, although there are likely to be a very
large number of different formats in any society, the
contradictions which occur are likely to be relatively few
in number, since the fundamental dilemmas are posed by the
different combinations of the basic elements to which I
referred earlier. Thus the solutions which are learnt in
one format will apply, more or less, to all those others
which embody a similar difficulty. Two basic contradictions have been considered in this monograph, and the
nullificatory methods noted here may be summarized as
follows (though, again, this is not to claim that these
lists are complete).

1 How may a superior criticize and correct the actions
   of an ideally good and competent subordinate?
   a by emphasizing the spotless future.
   b by treating the subordinate as ignorant and
      therefore guiltless in the past.
   c by proffering good excuses (thereby showing that
      the matter is something which needs excusing).
   d where reconstitutive work is considered essential,
      by letting the subordinates do the work themselves,
      i.e. by letting sinners name their own sins. (This
      is an extremely delicate time-consuming method,
      save where confession is institutionalized as in
      the Catholic Church.)
   e by passing such work to a subordinate.

2 How can authority be sustained when a subordinate has
   the right to question that authority?
   a by limiting severe dissent to the level of de-
      meanour, a tactic that is fine save where charac-
      ter-work is involved.
   b by leaving it to the superior to formulate his own
      incompetence and the inferior's disagreement, thus
      preserving the authority rule.

   c by the superior threatening to switch frame if the
      inferior tries to break frame.
   d by the inferior explicitly formulating challenges
      as non-serious (e.g. I don't know about this but
      ...).
   e by the inferior formulating challenges as coming
      from others, e.g. friends, colleagues and rela-
      tives.
   f by limiting a challenge so that it constitutes just
      a small section of the encounter, with an agreement
      to disagree and other normal business being trans-
      acted as before.
   g by switching between formats (as here between
      bureaucratic and clinical) though only on the
      superior's terms.
   h by the transformation of successful challenges into
      joint plans.

A rather different kind of nullification also needs
some consideration. Goffman tends to write as if there
was one and only one frame available for each activity-
system. He does indeed note how in any particular 'strip'
of action a person may engage in a series of different
activities, each of which has its own frame (Goffman,
1975a, p.561). He also notes how customers are often
portrayed in very different ways by service-providers when
they are alone in back-stage areas (1971a), thus contrasting the different frames which may exist for overt
and covert activities. But these are separate points. So
too is the argument that within any one frame, participants may make various copies or transformations of that
frame.

These things are not at issue. My concerns here lie
with 'basic' frames and not with their facsimiles, and
with just one activity-system, not with a sequence of
different systems or a contrasting pair.

As we have seen, there were a variety of ways in which
medical consultations could be framed. Moreover, in any
one encounter it was possible for more than one format to
be employed; a phenomenon which immediately poses the
question of how the reality of each format was kept
intact. Goffman treats the phenomenon of alternative
versions solely in terms of gaffes, mistakes, breaches and
asides - as a temporary slippage for which repair-work
might be necessary. But this is a quite separate matter.
The problem for staff and parents was: how could dual
versions of reality be maintained; how was it possible
for a clinical format to co-exist with the bureaucratic
format? (5) Once again the tactics used here may well

apply to other instances of twin framing and may be stated
in summary thus:
1 by the segregation of topic areas, reserving different
   formats for different topics.
2 by the segregation of participants, so that not all
   take part in every format.
3 by one format being given secondary status, e.g. by
   apologizing for its presence.
4 by bowdlerizing the contents of one or both frames –
   an extension of the rule of irrelevance.
5 by revealing the worthy aspects of one or both frames,
   i.e. by showing how each was important and might con-
   tribute to the other.
6 by turning it into a joke, an amusement for participants in the other frame.
   Finally, Goffman's analysis of the origins of a format
is distinctly limited. His account of the development of
situated roles sees the process as merely one of repetition (Goffman, 1961, p.96). (6) If the same activity is
played through often enough, then a stable ceremonial
order and division of labour simply emerges. A rather
more fruitful though equally brief suggestion is made in
'The Presentation of Self in Everyday Life' (1971a). Here
Goffman describes the ceremonial order of encounters as:

> ... a kind of interactional modus vivendi. Together
> the participants contribute to a single overall defi-
> nition of the situation which involves not so much a
> real agreement as to what exists but rather a real
> agreement as to whose claims concerning what issues
> will be temporarily honoured. Real agreement will
> also exist concerning the desirability of avoiding an
> open conflict of definitions of the situation. I will
> refer to this level of agreement as a 'working con-
> sensus' (Goffman, 1971a, p.21).

Such images point to a process of negotiation and
exchange as underlying role formats, even if this essentially political analysis is taken no further in
Goffman's own work. (7) We ourselves however may build
on this and, based on my reflections on the origins of
various medical formats, a number of points may be made
about the creation and re-creation of social forms.
   Let us start then with the model of ceremonial order as
essentially the product of political compromise between
the participants. Any one encounter is a social world in
miniature, whose outward form relies upon a miniature,
tacit contract. The shape that that contract takes is
largely the product of the particular interests and resources available to the participants.

At this point we must distinguish different levels of institutionalization. In one-off encounters the ceremonial order will be a fresh creation, but where the same activity-system engenders a number of routinely repeated encounters then, so long as the balance of interests and resources is perceived to be the same, the same overt form is likely to be repeated. Under these circumstances repetition may indeed result in institutionalization.

The possibility that one general solution will emerge is strengthened by two further considerations. First, a routinized solution to the problem of choosing a ceremonial order saves time, effort and worry. It diminishes uncertainty, cuts out initial skirmishing, avoids trouble and enables a rapid concentration on the task at hand. Second, as such a form enters general use, it acquires a moral as well as a political and technical force and becomes, not merely one way of solving things, but the way these things ought to be solved.

Given this institutionalization and its accompanying moral aura, role formats can become somewhat separate from the material interests that initially brought them into being. These little worlds can assume their own independent reality and status, set apart from the actions of their creators and re-creators. The original negotiation may have taken place many years, decades or even centuries ago, and current users may remain entirely unaware of the political and historical reality which they embody. (8)

This reification also enables a further kind of slippage. Since formats, once created, have an independent existence, they constitute a resource for all kinds of action. A form which has been invented to suit one set of purposes and interests may be used later on, under a different set of circumstances, to quite different ends. Something which started out as a rather deviant, daring use of a form may end up years later as the conventional means, the original usage having been forgotten.

Perhaps the most crucial aspect of this process of change is the gradual modification of one central element of the format: the rules that specify just when, where and with whom the format may be used. It is changes here that may permit the rest of a format to go relatively unchanged and yet be used in very different ways. A format that may have originated in and been intended for a highly delimited set of participants may become generalized throughout a population. Conversely, a form that was in general use may, over time, be restricted to a small minority of occasions or persons. In consequence, although the rules governing setting and membership are, at any one point, an essential part of a format, historically

viewed they may be seen as slightly to one side and separate from the rules formulating identity and action.

   One other major aspect of change may also be noted.
Under new circumstances, bits of an old format may be
combined with new elements, blending 'traditional' with
'modern' forms to create a new compromise. Indeed, all
formats must have their origins in this fashion, for none
can be created from totally new components. We build on
a stock of pre-existing forms and their elements, taking
bits from here and there and combining them as it suits
us. God may have created the world from chaos, the Earth
being without form and void, but the humbler products of
mankind are strictly secondary creations. The totally new
would lack both meaning and validity. Indeed it is the
very fact that forms are reified that lends them some
authority and weight. (9)

THE GENERAL INCIDENCE OF THE BUREAUCRATIC FORMAT

Having emphasized the importance of seeing role formats as
political products with a particular historical location
and set of uses, I now want to examine the bureaucratic
format in this light. Before I proceed to this, there is
one prior task. In deciding where to look for explanations it is essential to consider not just the nature
of the phenomenon but its incidence as well. If, for
example, the bureaucratic format is found only in medical
consultations with parents, then its origins are likely to
be different from the origins of a format that is used
with both parents and adult patients.

   As we shall see, although my own data relate solely to
children's clinics, there are quite good grounds for suggesting that the bureaucratic format, or something like
it, is a far more widespread phenomenon. In fact I shall
argue that this format, with one or two alterations, is
likely to be the predominant type of ceremonial order in
medical consultations within the National Health Service.
Its incidence within American medicine is more difficult
to estimate. There are no readily comparable American
studies that I know of, while the greater diversity of
types of medical service seems likely to produce a more
varied range of formats. Nevertheless, it seems likely
that it is at least a common mode of practice there,
perhaps the most common.

   In making these suggestions, I shall engage in two
principal moves. The first is to argue that although
medical work with children has some clear differences from
that with adult patients, there are some important in-

ternal devices, at least in outpatient consultations with
parents, through whose use the format can remain relatively unaffected by the presence of children. The second
move is to compare my own findings with those of other
studies conducted elsewhere within the British health
service. There are clearly not enough of the latter, nor
are they sufficiently detailed, for any definitive
statement to be made. What evidence there is does suggest
that the bureaucratic format, or something fairly like it,
is in standard use.

To see how children were excluded from the consultations we must first understand why this was done. The
reasons derive from the very special nature of children's
abilities and the equally special attributes which they
are granted by adults. (10) In brief, young children lack
even the most basic health knowledge. They do not necessarily know they are ill and may therefore lack any motivation to get better. They are also incapable of re-
porting on their illnesses in any precise fashion or of
co-operating with staff in any normal adult manner.

Rather than treating medical consultations in the
highly focussed manner of adults, young children create
their own meanings and activities out of the proceedings;
files, telephones and medical instruments can all be
turned into toys. Just as they lack an adult version of
the consultation, so too they lack a corresponding version
of themselves. Without an adult version of the future
they lack a self appropriate for medical work, for medicine is concerned with prognosis, prevention and care.

Given this incompetence, adults treat children in a
very special fashion. On the one hand, they are granted
some highly attractive qualities; they are, for instance,
seen as wonderful, amusing and innocent in ways that
adults cannot be (Davis and Strong, 1976b; Strong and
May, 1980). But on the other hand, they are given a
strictly subordinate status and placed under very tight
adult supervision.

It is this latter factor which explains children's
continued exclusion from consultations, even when they are
of an age to play some sensible part within it. At first
children are excluded because they cannot cope, save by
the use of an extremely inefficient, complex and time-
consuming mode - the game format (a mode whose use is
considered elsewhere (Davis and Strong, 1976a)). Later
on, they are excluded because their parents or guardians
still have the ultimate responsibility for their welfare,
while their own contributions are less skilled than those
of the normal adult.

This exclusion was no simple matter in the clinics

studied here. Since children were actually present in the
consultations, indeed their physical presence was normally
essential to the activity-system, they presented a
constant challenge to the smooth working of the adult
formats.

This dilemma was neatly solved by a judicious adult use
of whatever blend of competence and incompetence was possessed by a given child, though for descriptive purposes
it will be simpler to create two straw-children, the
'young child' and the 'older child'.

With younger children or with the mentally retarded,
adults turned their incapacity to focus on the consultation to their own advantage. Since children read other
meanings into events they were actively encouraged to do
so. Not only did many clinics provide toys, but staff
often gave them items of equipment to play with. The
child thus engaged, staff and parents could continue their
conversation undisturbed. Where there was an audience
present they were commonly expected to help out by playing
with the child - nurses, students and researchers all
having to muck in. Fathers, when they accompanied
mothers, often had this as their major role.

Children's exclusion from the main action was reinforced by the special qualities that adults attributed to
them. Just as parents spoke for children, they also spoke
to and about them in ways that adults did not speak of
each other, at least while in their presence. The
laughter and wonderment that might greet the actions of
young children were as much an indicator of their status
as incompetents as the open and routine criticism which
these might also earn. As incompetents they were clearly
subordinated to the adults present. Parents overtly and
continually instructed children on how to behave. They
warned them when they were going too far, rewarded them
for good behaviour, and punished them when they trans-
gressed.

Their character as incompetents was therefore publicly
established, indeed in clinics their character was public
property. Adults had majority rights not only in their
own characters but in those of the children present, and
examination of the latter was a common feature of clinic
work. Parents openly commented upon the sort of person
their child was, while they were regularly asked questions
about such matters, for many medical conditions commonly
had behavioural problems associated with them.

Young children themselves were obliged to play a part
in their exclusion from the adult conversation. Despite
their permitted engrossment in other activities, they were
expected to give due acknowledgment to the presence of the
main action.

If an adult encounter's integrity is to be maintained
in the presence of young children, a set of rules is
needed to govern the relationship to it of those bit-
players. Of these 'minimal encounter rules' the first
that children were expected to recognize was the obligation to acknowledge the beginning and end of the action.
Saying hello and goodbye was commonly expected of one-
year-olds and considerable time could be spent on getting
it right. Young children were also expected to recognize
the primacy of the adult encounter by dropping whatever
they were doing when required upon the adult stage. They
were also obliged to keep their own activities unobtrusive
- though considerable leeway was allowed here: by a
series of brief, infrequent and usually murmured comments,
many parents sustained an intermittent interaction with
their child, both pacifying it and yet paying some attention to the main encounter.

The fundamental principle that underlay all these procedures was that of adult authority. 'Because I say so'
was the implied rule that gave reason to events. In this,
adult-child interaction was marked, not just by an assumption of childish ignorance, but by a parallel and
equally basic rule of adult omniscience. Adults had
authority because they knew. Among adults such omniscience was often a matter for joking. Parents and
staff laughed at children's assumption that they would
know the answer to every why? and what? Yet such a
premise was fundamental to their interaction with
children. Most children took the fact of such authority
totally for granted and their revolts were transient affairs, rebellions not against the reasonableness of the
authority itself but against some minor edict. As such
they were treated as unimportant by adults. Young
children were not expected to recognize adult authority,
indeed their very incompetence might reasonably hinder
them in this. Their shyness, moodiness, their sudden
swings of involvement, all these might prevent obedience
to doctors' or parents' wishes. Besides, medical demands
were often novel and sometimes difficult or painful.

Given such incompetence, children's failure to observe
the medical conventions presented no serious threat to the
reality of the bureaucratic format. In other words, although the co-presence of two adult formats for the same
activity could present a severe challenge to the little
worlds which frames create, the presence of children was
a far less fundamental danger. The level of noise or the
constant interruptions might produce some technical difficulties, but the world in which young children lived was
of a clearly subordinate status and there was no need to
treat it with the seriousness accorded to adult frames.

Young children or the severely retarded could therefore
be readily excluded from most of the action, and even such
intrusion as they did make could be written off. But
older children possessed a much greater capacity to par-
ticipate sensibly in the consultation. What happened to
them? In fact, despite their larger abilities their exclusion was often yet more pronounced. The very powers
which might have given them a greater part than their
younger brethren were used against them. For such
children were now deemed old enough to obey adult authority fully. Allowances could be made for the very young.
They might even be given special activities to keep them
occupied. But older children were caught in a dilemma.
As children, they were subject to the fundamental rule of
childish incompetence and as such accompanied by an adult
representative who spoke for them. But as older children,
they were expected to stay excluded without any necessity
for effort by the adults; in other words, to have learnt
fully the minimal encounter rules required of subordinates.

Thus, beyond the age of five or so children were
expected to pay much greater respect to the social priority of the adult conversation. Good behaviour equalled
sitting quietly on a chair of their own, and pleasant
distractions were not provided. Children were now required to look as if they were ready and able to partici-
pate if called upon to do so; that is, some version of
adult demeanour was expected of them. But even for the
oldest children the call rarely came and when it did their
participation was closely supervised. Eleven- and twelve-
year-olds typically waited in silence while parents and
doctors discussed their case. Only exceptionally did such
children initiate topics and even then their participation
was still minor and treated in quite distinctive ways.

Since parents and others spoke for children they had
the right not merely to define what was in the children's
best interest but even to formulate their experiences,
that is to define what they had perceived, what they felt,
and how they would react to things. Their parents apparently knew them better than they knew themselves.
Their own versions of events were routinely overridden by
those who 'really' knew what the child had felt or would
experience. When older children were asked questions by
staff their parents often spoke for them, not waiting for
the child to answer. On such occasions children did not
fight back. They did not become angry and demand their
right to speak, for they had no such clear rights.
Indeed, to demand these might be taken by adults as a sign
of psychiatric abnormality, that one was not behaving as a

proper child. One eight-year-old seen at the Scottish
neurological clinic was being examined precisely because
of his failure to accept his subordinate status, and his
parents appealed to his behaviour in the clinic as yet
further evidence of this disturbance. (11)

Normally parents encountered no such difficulties.
Those from professional backgrounds might give their
children more scope to reply, but they too would frequently interrupt and cast doubt upon what had been said.
Doctors commonly gave older children a chance to talk, but
it was typically just the one chance. Even if taken it
lasted only a brief while; if not, the consultation
passed smoothly on to the parents.

In summary, children's incompetence and subordinate
status, when coupled with their acceptance of that status
and its sustained enforcement by adults, meant that they
could readily be excluded from large areas of interaction
and that consultations could take place principally
between staff and children's adult representatives.

This, of course, does not establish that the formats
used in this all-adult interaction are similar to those to
be found in consultations with adult patients, merely that
this is at least a possibility. The actual likelihood of
this occurrence can only be established through a comparison with studies of medical work with adults. But when
this is done it does seem as if something like the bureaucratic format may well be fairly uniform within the
National Health Service. Such an assertion is necessarily
tentative, since only a few other studies have gathered
extensive observational or taped data on medical practice,
while these researchers have had rather different aims
from my own. Nevertheless, certain striking parallels do
emerge between the principal format described in this
study and that which may be glimpsed in others.

There is at present no general study of consultations
in hospital outpatient departments, but there are two such
studies of general practice. Since general practice might
be supposed to differ far more from hospital paediatrics
than the latter differs from other kinds of hospital work,
such a comparison offers the thesis a severe test. Yet on
inspection there are certain close and vital similarities.
Byrne and Long (1976) is the most extensive study of medical practice so far undertaken, involving over 2,500 taped
consultations as conducted by 71 general practitioners, 60
of them British but including 5 Dutch and 6 Irish doctors.
Among their findings were these: doctors exerted almost
complete control over the interaction, so much so indeed
that the researchers did not think it necessary to take
patient variation into account when analysing individual

doctors' styles;   these styles were heavily routinized,
and in most cases minimized the amount of information
given to patients while allowing them little opportunity
to put their own point of view;   at the same time, most
patients seemed to be ascribed a reputable character.
Character-work, or as they term it 'chastisement' or
'negative behaviour', was 'comparatively rare':

> They (negative behaviours) do not commonly occur in any
> style with any degree of frequency. With the exception
> of a few consultations involving patients who were
> trying to extract drugs from doctors, or patients
> trying to have bottles of proprietary substances added
> to a prescription (e.g. Dettol), we have not been able
> to discover any evidence of a consistent negative style
> (Byrne and Long, 1976, p.161).

Further evidence comes from the observational part of
Stimson and Webb's study (1975) of general practice which,
though much smaller in scope, involving only 50 consultations and 5 doctors, was more directly concerned with
some of the matters dealt with here. They too note the
immense interactional power of doctors, though placing
some emphasis also on the patients' ability to negotiate.
Similarly, as in my own study, they note the way in which
appeal is made to a generalized body of medical knowledge
rather than to an individual doctor's competence. They
also discuss what they term the 'emotional flatness' of
medical consultations as well as their impersonality, and
remark upon the idealization of both medical expertise and
parental ignorance. They too emphasize the politeness
with which such affairs are conducted:

> There is rarely any conflict in the negotiation in the
> consultation. Both parties generally recognize and
> retain some semblance of formality and exercise
> restraint to prevent the encounter from completely
> breaking down ... verbal and non-verbal control strate-
> gies are often covert and rarely obvious or explicit.
> On the part of the patient particularly, they appear to
> operate beneath a facade of compliance and acquiescence
> (Stimson and Webb, 1975, pp.57-8).

Some central features of the bureaucratic format would
therefore seem to be found, not only in the Scottish
children's clinics which I studied, but in general
practice as well. This is not to say that every study has
a similar story. Research in some highly specialized
settings in Britain reports very different findings on one

of the most crucial dimensions of the bureaucratic format,
the moral character ascribed to patients. Two recent
studies of casualty departments (Jeffreys, 1974 and
Gibson, 1977) and a study of the work of a drug dependency
clinic (Stimson, 1978) suggest that in these settings at
least, and with patients such as drunks, drug addicts and
repeat drug-overdose cases, many doctors see overt character-work as a central part of the job. But these exceptions do seem to be exceptional. Elsewhere, on what
we know at present, it does appear plausible to argue that
the bureaucratic format, or something very like it, will
prove the standard ceremonial order within the British
National Health Service.

THE INFLUENCE OF CHILDREN UPON THE BUREAUCRATIC FORMAT

One cautionary note must be added. Even if the format is
used in many adult settings it is unlikely to take precisely the form delineated here. For, although child
patients can be excluded from medical encounters with considerable success, they do exert some influence upon the
interaction. In comparing the bureaucratic format that I
discovered in children's clinics with the descriptions of
the ceremonial order in general practice consultations, I
have picked out some things and omitted others. The
elements shared in common would seem to be these: firm
medical control; the idealization of both staff and
patients'/parents' character; an emphasis on service; a
combination of both politeness and impersonality; and an
emphasis on collegial rather than individual medical
expertise. However, there were other aspects of the
format that seem less likely to be found in medical work
with adults. Three things in particular need a mention,
all of which follow from the very different status accorded to children and adults.
    First, adults are normally responsible for their own
health, and medical professionals typically have no clear
rights to intervene if patients do not wish this, a position that is graphically expressed in the following
quotation taken from a study of general practice:

    Interviewer: Which raises another interesting question
                 about the extent of the doctor's responsi-
                 bility to patients. In that kind of case
                 where the patient says, 'I'm happy the way
                 I am,' there's damn all you can do about
                 it, I suppose?
    Doctor: There's damn all I *ought* to do about it.

Interviewer: If they want to kill themselves they
              should be free to do that.
Doctor: If he's free, white and over 21, that's my
        theory (Strong, 1980).

This may be an extreme statement but it expresses a
fundamental truth. Those who are of an age to take care
of themselves are normally allowed considerable freedom to
go their own way. By contrast, not only are children not
granted this right, but even those who are formally responsible for them, their parents or guardians, now have
to share that responsibility with the State and its
agents. Modern children are, at least in part, public
property.
    If this is so, why then should there be an alliance
rather than any more direct form of control? The answer
to this lies in the very limited exclusion of doctors'
practical authority. The extra responsibility placed upon
staff when they deal with children far outweighs the additional legal powers they are given. The law relating to
such matters is narrowly defined. It is not the case that
anything other than strict compliance with staff's instructions is either assault or alternatively neglect.
Parental action has to be extreme and a child's life in
some danger before staff appeal to the law. By and large
staff cannot force parents to do this or stop doing that;
they can merely suggest or imply. For although the state
claims some right to intervene in family life it does not
seek to supersede it. The ideal upbringing for a child is
thought to occur in the bosom of its family and the task
of the state is to support the family not destroy it.
Doctors have responsibility but not power.
    Thus, although there was an overt assumption in clinics
of a shared responsibility for the child, in practice
parents had most of it, as is clearly revealed in the
following quotation. In this consultation, the only occasion on which the ultimate responsibility for a child
was ever discussed, the child had presented with three
previous fits of an epileptic appearance; although the
hospital doctor advised that drug therapy should be
started immediately the parents rejected this, citing
their general practitioner's advice that this should begin
only if a fourth episode occurred. He had also apparently
said that it was their decision in the end; a statement
with which the doctor was forced to agree:

Dr J: Well, I can only advise you on things like
      swimming being properly supervised. It is your
      personal responsibility. So be it upon your own

head if you don't notify the school about
swimming or if you don't observe the rules about
cycling. All I can do is see her again in six
months' time. Now, have you any questions?
Mother: Well, don't think we're being ungrateful.
Dr J: Well, you're quite within your rights. It's your
responsibility. How you discharge it is your own
decision.

This incident also brings out another factor which con-
tributed to the making of an overt alliance between
doctors and parents. Such parental defiance was most
unusual and even here it was carefully warranted by appeal
to other expert opinion. Since staff still had access to
special legal powers, however rarely these were used,
parents were under greater constraints than those faced by
adult patients. Moreover, since they themselves were not
the patient, the sense of responsibility for someone else
was one which they shared with staff. In such circumstances it paid both parties to be accommodative.
There are, in addition, two other ways in which it
seems likely that the shared responsibility for a child
gave a distinctive flavour to the ceremonial order.
First, the universal idealization of parents' good character and the great lengths to which doctors went in main-
taining this may not be quite so strenuously followed in
some other medical settings. I do not mean by this that
investigative character-work with adult patients is likely
to be common, merely that staff's greater responsibility
for child patients, when coupled with their lack of power,
is likely to have made them especially nice to parents,
since they had few other resources on which to draw if
they wished to bend parents to their will.
At the same time the sharing of responsibility for a
child may also have lent the proceedings a rather more
uniformly serious tone than is normal in consultations
with adults. I have already noted the clinic's seriousness in this respect, but something more needs to be said.
Since it is up to adult patients to decide how to live
their own lives, they have some leeway in deciding how to
treat their illnesses. They can choose when or whether
they go to the doctor and, once they are there, they can
still make light of their complaints if they so wish.
Doctors in their turn can take their cue from their
patients and adopt a light-hearted approach, at least
where this seems appropriate. (12) By contrast, work of
some import which is done on behalf of someone else and
where that someone is small and defenceless may have a
more serious air. We may make light of our own suffer-

ings, indeed adults are normally obliged to (Goffman,
1972, pp.406-10), but the sufferings of little children
are another matter.

Finally, in considering the special qualities which the
bureaucratic format seems to have when used with child
patients and their parents, one should note that the
consultations I witnessed do not cover the entire range
of outpatient consultations. The restrictions on my data
are considered more fully in the introduction; but in
summary the study was limited to paediatricians and therapists and there are some grounds for arguing that such
staff may be especially considerate in their dealings with
parents, or at least this is what they themselves argued.
Indeed, every occupation claimed a special expertise in
this respect. They sustained this claim by each choosing
a different group for comparison. Health visitors contrasted their approach with that of local authority
doctors; local authority doctors and hospital therapists
compared themselves with hospital paediatricians; and the
latter distinguished their own approach from that of other
hospital doctors such as surgeons. Here for instance is a
paediatrician's analysis of the general orientation of
paediatrics:

> Dr I: There are two kinds of medicine ... this is very
> much a simplification ... there's the caring sort
> of medicine and the organizational sort of medi-
> cine at the other extreme. And each speciality
> is an admixture of the two, and I think paedi-
> atrics is well towards the caring end of the
> scale. It attracts people who are more inter-
> ested in the individual, more interested in
> families, more interested in the social side.

If this is so, then, although I would expect the format
to be the standard mode in outpatient clinics, it may well
vary in the delicacy of its application; though it must
be said that in terms of their overt idealization of
parents' character no important differences were observed
between the occupations studied here.

THE ORIGINS OF THE BUREAUCRATIC FORMAT: MEDICAL DOMINANCE

Having distinguished between the special features of the
bureaucratic format when used with children and those
which it seems to share with other medical consultations,
at least in general practice, we may now turn to consider
the origins of the more general form and the reasons for

its continued use. Formats are transitory things which
have no existence save in so far as they are reproduced
in individual encounters. What are the factors which have
led to the creation and continual re-enactment of the
central features of the bureaucratic mode across such
apparently wide areas of medical practice?

The method which I shall use in my answer to this
question is essentially comparative. Just as I have described other formats besides the bureaucratic in order to
highlight its main features, so here I will draw on the
rather different circumstances in which they occurred in
order to provide some explanation of the particular form
taken by the bureaucratic mode. I shall also make use of
various other historical and observational studies, for
these also may tell us something about the conditions
under which particular formats operate. The data on which
my generalizations are based are rather fugitive, but
enough has already been done to enable speculation by
other sociologists and I in my turn will add to this as
best I can.

In general, one can distinguish two broad strands
within the bureaucratic format which stand in need of
explanation. On the one hand there is the tight medical
control of the consultation, with the closely related
features of impersonal treatment and the appeal to collegial rather than individual expertise. On the other
hand, there are the idealization of the patient's character and competence; the ideal of service; the right of
patients to criticize that service, and at least the
semblance of rule by reason rather than by fiat. In considering medical practice sociologists in recent years
have followed Freidson (1970b) and emphasized the first of
these, that is 'medical dominance'. A more balanced view
must surely include the other and equally important
strand, that phenomenon which I shall term 'medical
gentility'.

Taking medical dominance first, its origins have
already been the subject of work of some merit and, while
it is pointless to repeat this at any length, it is worth
providing some details of the arguments here, since elements of them will play a major part in my own analysis of
gentility. Beginning then with Parsons (1951), he argues
that, compared with many other occupations, medicine has
certain special advantages in gaining power over its
clientele. This is an area where consumer judgment is
particularly ineffective, while the seeking of skilled
medical help means the intrusion of outsiders into intimate areas of one's life. In such matters the patient may
literally be naked and defenceless. Similarly Freidson

(1970b), despite placing a far higher emphasis on medical
dominance than Parsons, nevertheless concurs with his
basic explanation of the phenomenon – that of the great
asymmetry between medical and lay competence – although he
provides far more adequate documentation of his arguments.

Other writers however, while not dismissing these as
causes, have noted some further important matters. Their
method has been to place current forms of medical dominance in a more detailed historical and comparative
context and to contrast them, not just with medicine's
past, but with the situation that obtains in quite separate professions. Such a method has its problems, since
the factors cannot be held constant. One cannot really
compare the kind of technical expertise which doctors now
have with that which they possessed three centuries ago;
while the expertise possessed by lawyers or accountants
is of a quite separate order. Nevertheless, allowing for
these considerable difficulties, there do appear to be
several other factors which have played an important part
in determining the precise form taken by medical dominance. Johnson (1972) has argued that the degree of
control exerted by a profession over its clientele also
depends on the following conditions: the relative numbers
and financial resources of professionals and clients; the
extent to which the clientele form a group with homogene-
ous characteristics; the extent to which the clientele
are actually organized as a group; and the relative
social status of professionals when compared with their
clientele.

On his analysis, this explains why modern accountancy,
despite its considerable technical expertise, is dominated
rather than dominating. Accountants are dependent on a
relatively small number of powerful clients and to stay in
business must accommodate themselves to their demands. In
consequence many technical matters – such as how best to
introduce accounting methods which allow for inflation –
are ultimately decided by the clientele and not by the
profession. Jewson (1974) has pointed to a rather similar
situation in medicine. The relationship between doctors
and the aristocracy in eighteenth-century Britain was one
of patronage. Given their relatively greater resources,
such patients could enforce not just gentility but sub-
servience; doctors were granted no monopoly of technical
expertise, for aristocrats expected their own medical
theories to be taken into account.

On this kind of grounds, Johnson has argued that the
nineteenth century saw the creation of the modern form of
medical power, not simply because there was a major growth
in medical expertise at that time but because there was in

addition a parallel growth in a particular kind of client. He sees the origin of the modern profession of medicine as associated with

> ... the rise to power of an urban middle class which provided an expanding market for various services based largely on individual needs, whether private or entre-preneurial (Johnson, 1972, p.52).

This expanding bourgeoisie not only gave the financial support necessary for the employment of a relatively large number of doctors in a reasonable state of affluence, but also provided the material basis for medical domination. These doctors were members of a social class that was somewhat higher in status than many of their patients; and, in addition, although they themselves had grown in number, their patients had expanded at a far greater rate, were relatively varied in nature and were organized only at a family level. Faced with this relatively weak clientele, as well as themselves possessing a growing technical expertise, doctors could exert major control over the relationship with their patients.

So far, so good. But something more is necessary if we are to explain the particular form of medical dominance exhibited in the bureaucratic format. Just what this might be is best revealed by a comparison with the private mode. As will be remembered, the special quality of the latter was a concern for product differentiation: consul-tations were personalized; some time was taken over the individual requirements of each patient and parent; above all, the particular excellence of the individual doctor and his hospital was emphasized. The manner in which this was done might be constrained by professional rules and organizational demands, but nevertheless, since the patients could take their money elsewhere, the need to market a distinct product subtly influenced all aspects of the consultation. Personal touches paid.

By contrast, the bureaucratic format was rather more impersonal, gave less opportunity for parents to discuss matters with the doctor, and placed its emphasis on collegial rather than individual medical expertise. These properties would seem to derive from two factors: the rather smaller resources devoted to individual patients, and the deliberate restriction of competition between doctors. I shall consider both in turn.

The Scottish clinics catered for all, and aimed at giving the same standard of service to all. Given the volume of trade relative to the resources available, the most important commodity in clinics was time. Doctors

were normally in a hurry and in most settings impersonality and speed were a practical necessity. Given the
pressure of events, it was impossible for staff to engage
regularly in small-talk, to probe every anxiety, or to
answer every question in detail. Things were no different
in the American hospital. There too the normal format was
the bureaucratic; and the extra touches bought by private
patients were obtained only at the cost of minimizing the
time and thus the service offered to others.

This is not to deny that important changes might well
be possible within the brief time currently available to
medical practitioners. A little more information here and
there might do wonders. Nevertheless the constraints that
time alone imposes cannot be over-emphasized but are
rarely considered. (13) To make a comparison with
teaching: most thought about how to make teaching more
effective takes the size of school classes pretty much for
granted. This may be realistic but it leads us to ignore
the teachers' fundamental difficulty: how to control a
class of thirty children. Teaching might look very diffe
different if it could be done in classes of four. The
situation is much the same in medicine. The average
doctor within the National Health Service is obsessed with
time, and that obsession obliges him to control his
consultations as tightly as possible.

The other feature which gave the bureaucratic format
its distinctive shape, at least within the Scottish
clinics, was the set of severe restrictions on medical
competition. The general procedures here have been considered in chapter 2, but two points may need re-emphasis.
First, the system was divided so as to minimize the occasions on which competition could occur. There was a
careful division of labour, and the different parts tended
to complement each other rather than endlessly overlapping. There was only one hospital service, and although departments had their quarrels and demarcation
disputes none had a direct competitor. Since patients
could not refer themselves directly to the hospital it was
an adjunct to the services of the general practitioner
rather than an alternative. At the same time, some of the
normal motives and channels for competition were also in-
hibited. Since clients did not themselves pay for the
service, individual staff or agencies could not boost
their own income by attracting a larger or more profitable
trade. (14)

The absence of such incentives and opportunities was
central to the impersonal, highly controlled and relatively uninformative nature of the bureaucratic format. There
was, however, one potential flaw in this strategy of con-

tainment. Although patients had to register with just one
general practitioner and could only see other medical
staff, apart from local authority doctors, with the permission of this practitioner, they still had rights to a
second opinion. If parents were dissatisfied with the
verdict at the primary care level they could ask to see a
specialist. If they disliked his verdict they could ask
to see another specialist, and so on. Similarly, they
could register with a different general practitioner if
they disliked the one they had got. In principle, parents
had as much choice in the Scottish system as their private
counterparts did in the United States.

Here then, apparently, was a distinct threat both to
individual medical control and to the general policy of
collegial expertise. A little time needs to be spent on
explaining how it was circumvented. Once again, my argument here is based solely on what happened in the Scottish
children's clinics but it seems unlikely that things are
much different elsewhere in the British Health Service.

The first point to notice is that parents were kept in
relative ignorance both as to their rights and as to the
methods by which to gain a second opinion. Not only were
they not routinely informed that a second opinion was
available, but the general impersonality of clinics and
the basic rule of collegial wisdom meant that the inner
workings of medicine were never laid bare in the fashion
of the private format. Not much, of course, was necessarily revealed in the latter mode, but the very mention
of other doctors who had seen the child or were experts in
the area indicated that there were other named alternatives.

It also indicated, and this is my second point, that
there was nothing fundamentally wicked in parents' wanting
a second opinion, that it was an entirely reasonable thing
which any parent might want, and that the doctor would not
feel offended if this is what mothers chose. Finally,
since referral could come only through asking the doctor
one was currently seeing, to ask to be referred was a
risky business. Asking for a second opinion might preju-
dice one's present relationship with the doctor and give
one a bad name generally, something to be avoided in a
centralized medical service.

That parents might therefore be afraid to ask for
another doctor is brought out clearly in the following
example, one of the only two requests for a second opinion
witnessed during the study. In this case the paediatrician, Dr I, had previously discharged the child, although he was still attending the surgical clinic. However, the mother had written to Dr I saying that she

wanted to raise a number of matters with him;   and
thoughout this new consultation she discussed the child's
problem in a hesitant and embarrassed fashion.   Finally
she got round to the point:

Mother: Well, what I would like is ... (she broke off
       and paused) ...
Dr I: Would you like a second opinion about this?
Mother: Yes (said in a very gratified way).
Dr I: Have you spoken to Mr Blake (surgeon) about this?
Mother: No.
Dr I: (surprised tone) Why not?
Mother: Well, he seems very unapproachable. He didn't
      seem interested in Alistair. Although it could
      be as you say because it's too early to say yet
      (i.e. the child may be too young for proper
      testing), but as you think it's OK maybe we
      should leave it for the moment.
Dr I: Oh, no. Do have one if you want it. Shall I ask
      him for you? No ... (pause) ... that may not be
      quite such a good idea (everyone laughs). It
      might be best if you do it. Why not ask?
Mother: Won't he mind?
Dr I: Well ... (pause) ... No doctor *should* mind. ...
      What you've got to say is 'We're very worried,
      Mr Blake, and we'd be very willing to take him to
      anybody else as we're so worried about him.
      Could you please name somebody else whom we could
      take him to?' You see, I can't really name
      anyone, it's not my area.
Mother: You don't know anybody?
Dr I: Well, there are lots of doctors in Edinburgh who
      are very good. They're probably no better than
      Mr Blake but they're certainly good. But it's
      you who have to be satisfied, it's up to you.
      Mr Blake is the specialist in this area, he's the
      best man. I'm sorry I can't be of more help to
      you myself. I think it would be best if you say
      this yourself to Mr Blake. It would be best if
      it came through you.

For all her uncertainty this mother was middle-class,
as was the only other parent who asked for a second
opinion. What happened in this latter case shows with
considerable clarity the great power that gaining such
referral might give the brave. From being an impersonal
affair with every doctor interchangeable for most
purposes, the consultation might, in the right circumstances, be transformed into an area of personal and con-

flicting opinion and bear a closer resemblance to the
private than to the bureaucratic format. The following
quotations are from the consultation held just after the
mother's return from the English hospital to which she had
been referred when she asked for a second opinion:

> Mother: Dr Brown (England) said that this hospital (the
>   Scottish hospital) hadn't ruled out a heredi-
>   tary cause.
> Dr J: No, I'm sure he couldn't have said that. I'm
>   sure Dr McAllister (Scottish hospital) couldn't
>   have said that.
>
> Dr J: Quite frankly, the report from England is a
>   puzzle to us. What they say under the heading
>   'diagnosis', where they say they don't know,
>   differs from the bottom where they say it's ge-
>   netic and that there's a one in four chance of
>   its being passed on. Both Dr McAllister and I
>   can't understand how they can be so dogmatic that
>   it's genetic, and yet only place it in such a
>   vague diagnostic category.
> Mother: Well, I can't understand it. At the (English)
>   hospital, Dr Brown seemed right out on a limb.
>   He seemed definite, but no one else paid much
>   attention to him. Of course, when the news hit
>   me it was like a hammer blow, so I wasn't able
>   to take much in, but a registrar said to me not
>   to give up hope as Dr Brown was by no means
>   infallible. He treated me quite differently.

Having considered the particular conditions which
underlay medical control in the bureaucratic format, I
think it worth noting that the case I have just discussed
also has something to tell us about the more general phenomenon of the medical dominance. For this apparently
brave mother was by no means a typical patient. She herself was an ex-nurse while her brother-in-law was a
doctor;   and such behaviour, or something like this,
seemed relatively common among those with medical connections.
When discussing the idealization of staff's technical
authority, I noted that even those parents with some medical knowledge normally paid overt obeisance to this rule.
However, the proportion who covertly attacked the doctor's
authority was most striking. Apart from containing the
only mother to ask for a second opinion, this group also
held one of the few mothers to bring notes to a clinic,
and the only parent to actually make notes during a clinic

(though this latter action was merely reported of a previous occasion). Of the four mothers who made strong overt criticisms of the doctor, one was an ex-nurse and another a radiologist. In other words, although staff with medical connections or training made little direct appeal to their expertise, six out of the 19 such parents engaged in some of the most forceful action against staff's control of the consultation witnessed in the entire study.

This behaviour suggests that if the general run of parents had the knowledge that these others possessed, then the rules of the format would be quite different. Parsons and Freidson clearly have a major point when they emphasize the importance of technical expertise as a source of medical control, even if we ourselves must add to this the other factors which have been discussed in this section: relative status, relative numbers, the cohesion and uniformity of the clientele, the amount of time available, and the extent to which competition between doctors is encouraged or restricted.

THE ORIGINS OF THE BUREAUCRATIC FORMAT: MEDICAL GENTILITY

For all the reasons I have just given, doctors were able to exert a powerful control over the shape and content of medical consultations; a control which was particularly marked in the case of the bureaucratic format. And yet, as we have also seen, there were clear limits to their power. The practice of medicine necessarily involves systematic moral investigation and assessment, but it was only in the charity format that these concerns were made manifest. Elsewhere doctors went to great lengths to conceal the moral basis of their work and to transform medical practice into a neutral, 'scientific' affair that dealt with purely natural happenings. What resources did staff lack or parents possess that might account for the systematic idealization of parental character and competence? I have already noted that, at least in work with children, doctors were placed in a rather special situation. They were given considerable responsibility but little power, and were therefore obliged to adopt an accommodative strategy. And yet the idealization of the clients' character does not seem to be confined solely to the children's clinic, even if perhaps it is taken to extremes here. A more general explanation is therefore needed.

One answer to this problem has already been given by Parsons (1951), who is the only writer that I know of to have treated the phenomenon of medical gentility at

length. As we have already seen, he notes that patients
are in a rather vulnerable position, being ignorant as
well as ill. He then goes on to ask what prevents them
from being systematically exploited and why is it that the
doctor's relationship with the patient is characterized by
'universalism', 'functional specificity', 'affective
neutrality' and 'collectivity-orientation'. These rather
ugly terms cover somewhat different ground from my own,
since they are addressed not just to the ceremonial order
of medical consultations but to the whole doctor-patient
relationship. Nevertheless the matters that I have described, the rule of reason and the idealization of
character, would seem to be a part of the same package;
and the answers that he provides require careful examination.

In solving his puzzle, Parsons notes two important
characteristics of medical work in Western society; one
that is true just of modern times and the other that is
more universal. The first of these is medicine's establishment as an applied science. As a consequence he
holds that it shares in the universalistic values which
he sees as characteristic of science. The scientific
approach, on this ideal model, ignores the particularism
of status and social divisions and concentrates solely on
objective truths. It is therefore irrelevant to the
doctor-scientist whether he likes or dislikes his
patients, or whether they are rich or poor; these characteristics are simply not at issue. More generally, the
doctor, in whatever era, is faced with the difficulty that
medicine often deals in highly personal matters and involves potentially shaming acts such as physical examination. Delicacy and confidentiality are therefore
technically essential to the good practice of medicine;
or so he suggests.

There is clearly something in these two arguments, but
close inspection reveals that they alone cannot provide a
full answer. This failure is principally due to Parson's
inadequate phrasing of the question. The qualities that
he attributes to the doctor-patient relationship are far
from being universal even within our own society - as the
existence of the charity format makes clear. Thus the
general properties that he ascribes to modern medicine
cannot explain the major differences between one role
format and another.

Even if we treat these explanations as only a partial
influence, we are still faced with difficulties. Parsons
argues that medicine's role as an applied science serves
to guarantee the neutrality of doctor towards patient, but
he fails to note that this neutrality is often a spurious

construction. In other words, far from being neutral
because they are scientists, doctors can appeal to the
neutrality of 'natural' science in order to conceal the
systematic moral investigation and judgment in which they
are engaged. Finally, although he is surely correct in
seeing medicine as dealing with some matters which are
potentially shaming to any individual whatever his or her
culture, he fails to bring out the very special emphasis
on individual privacy and autonomy that is characteristic
of bourgeois culture.

I shall return to these points later. For the moment,
having seen that Parsons cannot offer us a fully adequate
explanation of medical gentility, it is worth considering
the location of the research on which his analysis was
originally founded. The consultations which he observed
and the doctors whom he interviewed were situated within
a system of private practice. As we have already seen,
such a system can enforce a highly personalized service
and is likely to go further still. The idealization of
patients in the private format is surely also, or at least
in large part, the product of competition between doctors.
Private patients might have little or no technical
knowledge, but they can certainly discriminate between
those doctors who are polite and attentive and those who
are not. To build or maintain such a practice doctors
have to establish goodwill and a good bedside manner is
an essential selling point. They might well feel like
moral denunciation on occasion but a sustained idealization of their patients' character is the only guarantee
of a thriving business.

If anything, this tendency is likely to be reinforced
by the achievement of a legal monopoly of practice and the
profession's code of ethics, for these place limits on the
extent to which competition is explicitly based on different theories and techniques, and tends to concentrate it
instead on the smooth delivery of service.

Here then is the key to the idealization of the private
patients. But why should this same phenomenon be found in
a context where competition between doctors is systematically excluded? If the bureaucratic format is, as it
were, robbed of the more personal touches of the private
mode, why should it not also lose that heavy emphasis on
the moral worth and competence of the patient?

My answer to this is that the power given to patients
under a system of private practice can be replaced by
another kind of resource. The power of the consumer
within the British Health Service is exerted not through
direct payment but through political means via the mediation of the state. As Navarro has written:

It is impossible to explain the creation of the NHS
without understanding the relationship of class forces
in Britain and the war-time radicalization of the
working class that had called into question the
'survival of capitalism'....   Indeed, labour movements
have historically viewed social services (including
health) as part of the *social wage,* to be defended and
increased in the same way that *money wages* are.   In
fact, Wilensky has shown how the size of social wages
depends, in large degree, on the level of militancy of
the labour movements (Navarro, 1977, p.286). (14)

In other words, polite medical service can be the
product of a trade-off between organized labour and
capital and may be bought through political as well as
financial muscle. In this situation doctors are still
dependent upon their patients' good will, but in a
somewhat different manner. Since they are not paid
directly by the individual, and since medicine here is a
less competitive business, doctors are not so constrained
to provide a personalized service. But because the financial position, prestige and degree of self-control of
the profession as a whole are under direct political
management and are themselves a political issue, it pays
doctors to be polite to the great mass of their patients.
In consequence there are strong collegial pressures for
politeness to all, pressures that are reinforced as well
as exemplified by the creation of a uniform national
service.
In discussing medical dominance I noted Johnson's argument that a certain degree of heterogeneity among their
patients fosters professional control. However, he goes
on to note that major social and financial divisions among
the clientele may fragment the profession, producing quite
separate types of service in which practitioners may
develop quite separate sets of interest in the struggle
for resources. By contrast, where a national health
service is created, doctors have a set of joint interests
in common and there will be strong pressures for the
development of a common culture: a culture in which
gentility and service to all patients receives a heavy
ideological emphasis - so long at least as working-class
patients retain some political power. Crucial elements of
the private format are therefore retained despite the abo-
lition of direct payment and of most competition between
doctors. (15)

THE VICTORY OF BOURGEOIS MEDICINE

One other way of putting all this is to note that the
British National Health Service, despite the fairly radical shift in power on which it was based, retains a fundamentally bourgeois flavour - a proposition whose truth
cannot be fully grasped unless one stands back a little to
consider the rules for the entire 'doctor-patient relationship' of which the bureaucratic or private formats
are merely parts:

1 Doctors serve the individual client, their duty
towards him is both compelling and undivided, they should
serve no other. This principle is of course modified in a
number of ways, for instance as regards sick notes, research, insurance examination, and the care of the incompetent, whether children, the insane or the geriatric;
nevertheless, it remains the basic orientation of medical
practice.

2 Given the stress on the professional's service to his
or her client, there is a central ethical emphasis on the
confidentiality of the relationship. That is, not only is
the relationship solely between doctor and patient and for
the benefit of that patient, but the transaction is
private and to be kept secret from others. Once again
some practical modification may be made for students,
other staff or for researchers, but the principle still
holds.

3 Just as the doctor serves the individual client, so
patients typically belong to individual doctors, and the
relationship between different doctors and a particular
patient is subject to a delicate professional etiquette.
When a general practitioner refers a patient to a hospital
specialist that patient is still his, and he has the right
both to receive regular reports from the specialists and
to reject those reports if he so wishes. Scottish local
authority doctors, since they owned no patients, had no
right to treat and had to refer to other professionals
for this.

4 Not only is medical service given in a confidential
fashion by specific doctors to specific individuals, but
individuals in many important respects also choose the
service they receive. The range of choice of practitioner
may be restricted in a national health service or a pre-
payment plan, but the principle of consumer choice is
still central. Fundamentally, it is the clients themselves and not medical personnel who normally decide when
they should seek treatment and have advice. Freidson
(1961, p.197) and Stimson and Webb (1975, p.155) have
argued that since doctors have a monopoly of many crucial

types of medical resource and a virtual monopoly of medical knowledge, this choice is necessarily limited. However, despite the state's granting of legal rights to
practice, doctors have received no equivalent powers to
enforce that practice on their patients. Adults cannot be
brought to court for self-neglect, and when most doctors
think of the law they think of their own rather than their
patients' possible malpractice.

5 Patients have these rights because, like economic man
in classical economics, they are overtly assumed to be
rational, knowledgeable, competent and properly motivated.
As such they will themselves typically recognize when they
are ill and will wish to alter this state by taking or
seeking appropriate care.

6 Medicine is an enterprise which deals primarily with
natural phenomena. (This too has its parallels with
classical economics, which gave large areas of bourgeois
theorizing the status of natural laws.) This reification
of illness has two consequences. First, since the state
deals primarily with social matters it has little business
in medicine. It may intervene to ensure that services are
properly organized or that treatment is available to all,
but the conduct of medicine itself is essentially a matter
for those who specialize in the ways of the natural.
Second, since illness is a natural affair, patients' moral
character is in no way questioned by it. Medical inquiry
is concerned not with the investigation and rooting out of
personal dereliction but with the clinical analysis and
treatment of the biological sphere.

Here then, with its emphasis on the primacy of the
individual and its vision of the doctor-patient
relationship as essentially a private contract, is a
distinctively bourgeois conception of medical encounters.
(16) Yet, as we have seen, there is no necessary reason
why the doctor-patient relationship should look like this.
Indeed, under other conditions, keeping well, far from
being a private concern, might be regarded as an essentially public duty. Instead of patients seeking
treatment on their own initiative and having some right to
determine whether or not they are ill, they might indeed
be sought out and then treated, regardless of their own
wishes. Rather than emphasizing the privacy and confidentiality of medical transactions, these might well be
matters of public record and humiliation. Far from being
an overtly natural and neutral phenomenon, medicine might
be transformed into a thoroughly moral and judgmental
activity. Such a vision has been most thoroughly captured
in Samuel Butler's 'Erewhon':

If a man falls into ill-health, or catches any disorder, or fails bodily in any way before he is seventy
years old, he is tried before a jury of his countrymen,
and if convicted is held up to public scorn and
sentenced more or less severely as the case may be.
There are sub-divisions of illness into crimes and
misdemeanours - a man being punished very heavily for
serious illness, while failure of eyes or hearing in
one over sixty-five, who has had good health hitherto,
is dealt with by fine only (Butler, 1977).

'Erewhon' may be nowhere, but elements of its laws can
readily be found somewhere. Groups with little political
or financial power and of a degraded social status have
often been treated in very different ways from their more
fortunate brethren. The degradation that this may inflict
is readily compatible with the loftiest ideals of service.
To take an instructive example from outside medicine, the
middle-class Evangelical reformers of Victorian Britain,
while equally critical of the morals of all classes of
society, used quite separate means to ensure their reform.
The middle and upper classes were to be persuaded by argument; the lower required laws (Bradley, 1976). Similarly, health visitors were, and in some respects still are,
a kind of health police, enforcing medical 'law' upon the
lowest social classes (see Dingwall, 1977).
    Again this division almost exactly parallels the split
between the charity format and the other model described
in this study. The doctor who used the charity format was
as concerned as any of her colleagues with the health and
welfare of the poor, and also (Parsons might note) laid
far greater overt stress in her consultations on the
scientific aspects of medicine than any of them. Yet as
we have seen there was little trace of gentility in most
of her medical consultations and they provide a graphic
example of a distinctly non-bourgeois version of medical
practice. (Or rather they reveal what may happen to some
patients when bourgeois norms are applied solely to the
bourgeoisie.)
    For her, an individual's ability to pay for medical
services was based on moral characteristics; anyone who
worked hard and lived sensibly could normally afford
private care. The mothers at the clinic were therefore
suspected to be either morally or rationally deficient,
or indeed both. (17) This philosophy gave the doctor a
mandate to investigate all aspects of their lives; for
her task was not simply the treatment of illness but the
reform of the poor so that they had no need of such
charity in the future. Such investigation served a

further purpose also, for it helped to distinguish the deserving from the undeserving, cases of genuine hardship from those who were lazy or evil. A charity service, in a country where medicine normally had to be paid for, not only aided those who had fallen on hard times through no fault of their own but might also, on this theory, be abused by those who were well capable of bettering themselves if they had a mind to.

We may also contrast the medical fate of those who live in total institutions or totalitarian societies with those of the freer sick elsewhere. At the height of Stalin's production drive doctors were issued with quotas for the numbers allowed to be ill; once these were filled no one else could fall sick (Waitzkin and Waterman, 1974). By contrast, it now appears that some political offences may be re-cast as psychiatric illness within the Soviet Union. (18) Armies, prisons and mental hospitals may similarly place drastic restrictions on individuals' right to be or not to be ill, choosing themselves what is to count as illness and when and how it is to be treated.

To draw a moral from all this: it is currently fashionable to see the National Health Service as representing only a partial victory for the working class. But the consideration of what a fully social system of medicine might mean shows just how partial such views are. For all our sophistication there is a strong temptation to assume that the bourgeois version of medicine, far from being the product of specific historical circumstances, is the only way in which these matters could be dealt with. Freidson (1970a, p.214) has noted how Becker, when writing of deviance, excludes biological illness as beyond the sociologists' remit. Similarly, other writers, including Freidson, take for granted the assumption that the doctor-patient relationship is and should be a private contract (using 'private' in the sense of privacy). The things which make sociological news are the exceptions to this principle: the fact that, despite the individual's right to choose or reject treatment, there is also a social duty to keep fit and co-operate with expert advice - a sick role; or the fact that although doctors claim to serve the individual patient they may sometimes in practice oppress her.

Bourgeois freedoms deserve a mention in their own right; and the fact of their continuation - in only slightly modified form and in quite different historical circumstances from those which led to their creation - needs its own analysis. Johnson (1972) has noted how the National Health Service represents merely a partial mediation by the state which now determines who should get the

service, but is not directly concerned with the manner of
its delivery. He himself represents this as a victory for
the profession, which can continue its old dominance un-
checked. Looked at in another way, the Health Service,
for all its defects, is a major triumph for the patient
too. He or she can now get a standard of care that before
was available only to the wealthy and, at the same time,
can retain many of those same rights to polite treatment,
privacy and choice that were previously guaranteed only by
private practice. And things might not have been so.
Patient power is the only sure road to medical gentility.

POLICY CONSIDERATIONS

I shall now conclude with some reflections on the possible
implications of my analysis for the current practice of
medicine. Because my comments have been fairly abstract,
my remarks here will be equally general, although I do
have one or two specific things to say on occasion. Since
I cover a variety of topics, most of which are uncon-
nected, I shall merely list the points I wish to make.

   1 The presence of students in clinics had a major
effect upon the shape and content of interaction with
parents, and this was so even where no overt teaching was
done. This system may produce the worst of both worlds.
Not only did parents get less time, less privacy and an
atmosphere which might make their lay remarks look 'silly'
(at least to them), but teaching was also affected. I can
make no proper assessment of the effectiveness of teaching
by such a method, but the concern of staff to minimize the
impact of students on patients placed major restrictions
on what could be taught. Doctors were put in an impossible dilemma: those who worried a lot about teaching
squeezed the parents out, while those who worried about
the parents never taught, and the students just sat there,
quietly bored. There were some doctors who could not cope
at all with the conflicting demands and whose clinics resembled a three-ring circus run by a dazed but frantic
ringmaster. Other methods of teaching might well prove
more satisfactory to both patients and students.

   2 The doctors in this study overtly defined medical
work as a 'natural' phenomenon. In one example with which
I have dealt 'psychiatric' matters were normally avoided
and doctors concentrated instead on the purely organic.
That this avoidance is not an idiosyncrasy of paediatricians is shown by McDonald and Patel's (1975) study of
Glaswegian psychiatrists. Even they apparently preferred
organic to functional complaints. These preferences are

scarcely surprising given the heavy emphasis on the
organic side in medical training; the firm rule that a
patient's character is to be overtly idealized; and the
extremely circuitous and time-consuming work that is
involved if patients are to be both criticized and idealized - whereas doctors have relatively little time for
each patient.

The reification of illness that results from this
avoidance has a central consequence for medical work. In
our bourgeois world patients have certain rights to define
themselves as physically ill, regardless of doctors'
covert medical opinion. (Even parents who must share
their responsibility for a child still have important
powers here.) These rights are, of course, aided by the
fact that many things which may be social in origin can
have organic consequences. Tension at work or at home may
lead to vague pains, headaches, ulcers, enuresis and so
on. In other words the reification of problems within the
ceremonial order of the clinic is often matched by a quite
literal reification of problems within the body of the
individual patient.

The challenge which this double reification presents to
many branches of medicine is considerable. Although many
doctors, or at least those considered here, are often
content to ignore it there are some who feel that this is
shirking their professional duty; the proper doctor
should seek to go behind the presenting complaint and
uncover the 'real' problems (Balint, M., 1964; Balint E.
and Norell, 1974; Byrne and Long, 1976).

Whether doctors are the appropriate people to engage in
this is a vexed question, and important objections can be
raised to their doing so (Stimson, 1977). I myself will
mention just one problem posed by these attempts to produce a more thoroughly social version of medicine.

To transform one's problems into illness should not, I
think, always be seen as an evasion which must be faced up
to. Precisely because of its natural status, illness can
offer escape from difficult situations and thus soften the
edges of a harsh world. To remove this freedom from individuals without having any better alternative to put in
its place is a brutal act.

If doctors were always to investigate the social
reasons behind the natural appearance, they might well
lose half their practice. From the position of bourgeois
ideology, one of the great advantages of doctors is that
most of them do not normally want to poke around in the
patient's psyche (though women suffer more in this
respect). Going to the doctor is, on this version, a
straightforward transaction. The patient presents the

problem and the doctor deals with it if he or she can.
But go to a psychiatrist or a social worker and who knows
where you will end up? (19)   If ordinary doctors ever use
psychotherapy in a big way many patients might never
present themselves at all.   Who knows what might be
'found' behind even the most natural-seeming illness? (20)

At present this possibility seems remote.   The real
alternative to bourgeois medicine is more likely to come,
not from the doctors themselves but from the social
workers, who in Britain at least are attached in ever-
increasing numbers to medical institutions and to whom
such problems may increasingly be referred. (21)

3 As I have argued, patients can not only choose to be
ill – within limits – they can also choose not to be ill,
or at least most adult patients can.   When they are not
ill doctors have almost no purchase on them at àll.
Health is no business of doctors, only illness.   It is
this, coupled with medical gentility, that renders the
ordinary doctor's participation in preventive medicine a
rather unlikely event.   To engage in systematic reform of
the way we live – what we eat, drink or smoke, how we
bring up our children;   these are affairs beyond the
doctor's normal remit, unless, that is, they result in
clear illness.   There may well be exceptions to this rule,
but the principle at present stands firm.   Doctors have
not the time, the training, the inclination or the warrant
to intervene routinely in patients' lives.   Once again,
the currently fashionable doctrines of a more thoroughly
social medicine place a much greater emphasis on prevention than has been common in recent years.   As things
stand, however, it seems unlikely that most doctors can
take much part in this movement.

4 If the causes of the impersonality, lack of choice,
and relatively uninformative nature of the bureaucratic
format are lack of time and an absence of competition,
then the only way to amend these, if that is what is
wished, is to devote far more resources to national medical services.   And yet the issue has rarely been faced.

To take one example, Horobin (1978) has shown how the
norm set for the size of general practitioners' lists
within the Health Service, perhaps the most fundamental
determinant of a doctor's work, has been the subject of
almost no political or academic discussion.   It seems to
have been derived simply by dividing the population by the
number of general practitioners practising at the time the
service was created.   Fierce debate has occurred over the
areas which are over- or under-doctored according to this
norm and what might be the best policies to correct this;
whether or not the norm is desirable in the first place
has rarely been at issue.

I noted earlier the strong similarities with education
in this respect. The way in which the norms of class or
practice size are taken for granted is also illustrated by
the great media scares that occur every now and again due
to demographic and student change. The fuss over whether
we are producing 'too many' teachers or doctors is all
based on the largely unexamined assumption that our
current ratios represent an ideal standard. Similarly,
the efforts to produce a better service all concentrate on
modifications which leave this norm untouched. Teachers
discuss the pros and cons of new types of teaching and
assessment, whether to abolish exams, or teach by projects
instead of essays. Doctors are supposed to develop a more
'person-oriented' style or else get more para-medical
assistants. Meanwhile teacher-pupil and doctor-patient
ratios stay pretty much the same.
    Far more research and discussion is therefore needed
about the differences produced in medical consultations by
simple variations in their length. Unless one is fully
aware of the constraints which time imposes, any discussion of the doctor-patient relationship takes on a
curiously abstract air quite remote from daily experience.
    5 Having said all this, I must take care not to be
misunderstood. The argument that the bureaucratic format
is rather more controlled and impersonal than the private
mode is quite separate from the judgment that this is a
bad thing which needs an immediate remedy. Even if it can
be convincingly shown that more resources do in fact produce a more personalized service, it is not clear that
this should have any priority, at least as a general aim.
It can be argued that many of the personal touches which
seem to be added by competition are of a somewhat spurious
nature.
    As I have argued elsewhere (Strong, 1979), there is a
distinct tendency within sociology to treat medical
matters in much the same way as do soap-operas, investing
them with enormous significance and turning the most
routine treatment into human drama. There is clearly good
reason for this on occasion, but as a general outlook it
can be misleading. Many consultations are mundane affairs
in which patients are willing to tolerate impersonal
treatment in return for help of some kind. Besides, it is
not as if this is anything unusual. To understand medical
service fully we must see it as just one of a great many
impersonal relationships into which consumers must enter
in our society: doing the shopping; buying a house;
selling a car or seeing the doctor are all, in
Wenglinsky's phrase, errands (1973; Strong 1977a). What
customers are most interested in here is competent and ef-

ficient service, and they are quite prepared to sacrifice
the more personal touches if this is the price they must
pay. Few grocers have survived the supermarket era.
   The crucial issue then turns around the technical
quality of the service that is offered; and on this
matter I am not competent to pass judgment although, as I
noted in the introduction, there is no evidence that I
know of that the medical care offered patients in the
bureaucratic format was inferior to that found in the
private format.
   What I can say is that private practice certainly
fostered the impression that the technical quality of care
was something special. This appearance of excellence was
based, ironically enough, on parents' very scepticism
about medicine. Although most patients have some general
distrust of doctors, they typically lack the expertise to
pass correct technical judgments on the wisdom of any one
doctor. Nevertheless they still try to assess staff's
competence as best they can. In a competitive market
doctors can exploit this weakness by explicitly fostering
the delusion of customer wisdom. The private-practice
style observed in this study was one in which the doctor
subtly indicated his own individual merit, flattered
patients by treating them as particularly promising medical students, and congratulated them on having chosen so
well. The personal charm, the lavish use of technical
terms (displayed in the guise of enabling patients to make
a better choice), the routine battery of impressive though
often useless tests, and the casual mention of colleagues
in famous hospitals, all 'prove' that you cannot get
proper medicine unless you pay for it; a proof that seems
to have taken in a surprising number of American sociologists. Or perhaps this is not so surprising if one re-
members that thinking oneself an artful consumer is such a
cherished identity in the games the middle classes play.
   6 Despite the absence, as I would see it, of any
general need for a highly personal medical service, there
are many instances where something rather better than the
standard bureaucratic package is desirable. In particular, relatively impersonal treatment may be fine for many
acute or trivial ailments, but is far less so for chronic
conditions. Where a whole way of life is involved then
ten, fifteen or, if the patient is lucky, thirty minutes
seems rather inappropriate. The parents of the handicapped children in this study did get more time than most
others and did, as we have seen, get a somewhat more
personal service. Even so, it scarcely matched the complexity and scale of the problems which they faced. (22)
   Securing a better service here is not just a question

of devoting more resources to those most in need. It is
also a question of staff's attitude. It is not simply
that the bureaucratic format is best suited to acute conditions, but that doctors themselves tend to prefer acute
medicine. Trained to cure and deriving great satisfaction
from the speedy solution of organic problems, they are
constantly faced with patients for whom they can do little
and whose difficulties are as much social as natural.
Their normal reaction to this dilemma is to shy away from
it, one that in some respects may be no bad thing, as I
have argued. There are, however, contexts in which their
special skills could be put to much greater use than
occurs at present, at least on the evidence presented
here.

One such circumstance stood out clearly in this study,
and it is with this that I shall end. Doctors believed,
and there was a good deal of evidence to support their
belief, that the parents of handicapped children were
often racked by a feeling of personal guilt, a feeling
that they themselves were responsible for their child's
condition. And yet, as we have seen, doctors did very
little to help such parents. The search and destroy
methods used for trivial anxieties were not employed here.
Parents, or so it seemed, were afraid to reveal their
fears, doctors were afraid to search for them.

This mutual avoidance of the matter may be intelligi-
ble, but there is surely no necessity for things to be
this way and every reason why they should be otherwise.
For here at least doctors can offer some practical help.
They may lack cures but they can give comfort. Moreover,
it is a comfort which only they can properly provide.
Social workers, where they are available, may have the
training and the time to investigate the parents' world;
but only doctors can pronounce with any authority on the
likely etiology of a child's condition, only they can cast
things firmly within the natural sphere. (23)

9 A methodological appendix

The subject of this book concerns those rules which make up the bureaucratic format; but finding rules in inter- action and, more especially, keeping them alive in cap- tivity so that others may see them too, presents consider- able difficulties. A brief account of these difficulties and of the various ways of tackling them may therefore be necessary, at least for the sceptical or technically- minded reader.

The method of data collection used in this study was primarily based on observation. Observation, or the systematic recording of behaviour, has several advantages over interview data in the study of social rules. First, interviews are no guide to actual behaviour (Cicourel, 1964; Phillips, 1971). Many of the studies of doctor- patient relationship, since they are based solely on interviews, are purely accounts of attitudes. As Stimson and Webb's (1975) study has shown, there is no necessary relationship between what patients do in medical consul- tation and what they say they do in another context. (In group interviews women recounted heroic tales of their personal combat with their doctors, but no such behaviour was actually observed in GPs' surgeries.) What people say depends very much on what questions are asked, who asks them and the general sense of the occasion. Even where rules are accurately recounted – and interview methods allow no clear check on this – it is still impossible to determine how such rules relate to actual behaviour. For no rule specifies the grounds of its own application. That is, to use a rule one also needs a further set of rules to say when, how and in what circumstances the rule is to be used. These rules of thumb are rarely spelt out formally, save in legal proceedings. Aside from these difficulties, there are good grounds for arguing that people are incapable of immediate recall of many aspects

of their behaviour. It is not merely that our accounts
are guided by our prejudices or immediate circumstances
but that we fail to notice much of what we do, for we
attend only to those things that concern us most. As
Fingarette (1969) has argued, there is no need for us even
to be conscious of following a rule in order to actually
do so. Interview data therefore contain a strong bias
against the routine and the non-eventful.

The strategy that was followed in this study was
therefore to observe and record the behaviour in question
systematically and then to engage in detailed analysis and
exemplification. This has certain advantages for both
researcher and reader. For the researcher it provides a
source of data which, unlike pre-coded material, is independent of the analysis and can therefore be re-read or
re-played as a check against that analysis. Similarly,
in so far as examples of data are provided in the text
they provide readers with the possibility of independent
checking.

Certain difficulties still remain. The method is
highly labour-intensive and thus, like informal interviewing, does not permit of ready generalization, though
this difficulty may be surmounted if other comparable
studies are available (Becker, 1969a). More crucially,
there are major problems involving the accuracy of note-
taking, the detection of rules in observed interaction,
the quantification of such phenomena, the influence of the
observer upon the recorded material and the general difficulties of analysing qualitative data. Each of these
matters deserves some attention.

RECORDING INTERACTION

There is a variety of procedures for recording interaction, each with its own advantages and disadvantages.
Audio or video-tape offer the possibility of highly accurate recording but are obtrusive and pose major problems
for transcription. The pen and paper method used in this
study is, by comparison, extremely inaccurate; much that
is spoken is lost and much that is recorded is no doubt
altered. At the same time however, it does enable the
relatively easy study of a very large number of cases and
it is this which justifies its use in the present study.
To have transcribed and analysed a mechanical recording of
over 1,100 consultations, some of them up to an hour long,
would have been a forbidding task and yet, unless one had
gathered some such large body of data, there would have
been an insufficient number of 'deviant cases' for analy-

sis - and as we have seen it is the exceptions which prove the rule.

Moreover, this rather crude method of recording seems relatively tolerable for the somewhat gross matters with which I am here concerned. To illustrate the broad components of a role format, one does not require the same degree of accuracy in recording as is necessary for those concerned with the minutiae of conversational analysis, where the precise sequence and phrasing of word and gesture is essential to the analysis.

QUANTIFYING QUALITATIVE DATA

My central assumption here is that it is illegitimate to attempt to count social phenomena more precisely than lay persons are themselves able to. (1) An examination of everyday counting practices soon reveals that the kind of things which human beings are able to count with any ease, and in which they may reasonably expect others to arrive at a similar total, are remarkably limited. They belong solely to the world of objects. We count cars, meals or bathrooms, but counting actions or emotions seems to be a much trickier business. To say, 'I had a good day,' is a meaningful statement but to attempt to quantify its good aspects in any precise fashion is not possible. (2) Under inspection, 'good' things have their 'bad' side too; every silver lining has a cloud. In consequence it would be entirely bogus to quantify many aspects of the data which I have described here. Nevertheless, following Douglas (1971), I think there can be an important degree of certainty over people's typical meanings. Indeed, organized life would be impossible if this were not the case. A limited version of counting is thus often possible, using quantificatory statements such as 'always/typically/rarely/never'.

The reader will therefore have found a mixture of kinds of quantification within the book. On some matters, for example the number of foster-mothers or cases seen in a clinic, I feel able to be precise. For many other matters which deal with actions rather than objects and where far more judgment is therefore necessary, 'typically' or 'rarely' seem more sensible terms. For a few kinds of action I have in fact used numbers. Where these were extremely unusual and I had only a limited number of cases to study, it seemed reasonable to risk a little more quantification. Since these cases could be analysed in considerable detail, terms like 'three', 'four' or 'five' have sometimes been used. I cannot really claim to know

that there were exactly three, four or five instances of
X or Y. I have used numbers here because these were
highly infrequent happenings for which I was specifically
searching, and any possible examples of which had been
given a good deal of thought. Such numbers also have, I
confess, a rhetorical significance. 'Look, I could only
find five!' sounds more convincing than 'I found very few
exceptions'.

THE INFLUENCE OF THE OBSERVER

One objection that is commonly made to studies such as
this is that although observation is undoubtedly a more
direct way of studying action, the presence of the observer changes the action in a way that interviewing does
not. Since all action is oriented in some way to the
immediate social context, it is undoubtedly true that the
fieldworker changes that situation. However, there are
good grounds, at least in the present study, for arguing
that such effects were minimal. First, as Becker has
emphasized, the daily business of life has to get done,
and in clinics there was no other time or place for it to
be done:

> The people the fieldworker observes are ordinarily
> constrained to act as they would have in his absence
> by the very social constraints whose effects interest
> him; he therefore has little chance, compared to the
> practitioners of other methods, to influence what they
> do, for more potent forces are operating (Becker,
> 1969b, p.43).

Second, such a presence was by no means strange. The
medical settings that were studied here were highly public
places with nurses, students, other staff and sometimes
other patients all watching the action or overhearing
parts of it. Fieldwork was not uncomfortable since there
were so many others engaged in somewhat similar activities. Thus, staff rapidly became used to the presence of
researchers and treated them as part of the furniture.
Some of them indeed, despite being told otherwise, seemed
to think that only the patients were being studied.
    As for the clientele, it must be remembered that all of
what they said was for the record, regardless of the
record made by the researchers, for doctors themselves
routinely made notes on what was said by parents during
the consultation. It is quite likely that had there been
no audience and no note-taking at all, conversations might

have taken a somewhat different turn. Parents might have
found 'personal' and emotional matters somewhat easier to
raise, and they could well have felt more relaxed and been
more informal. However, such constraints were in the
nature of the settings, they were not imposed upon them by
the research.

UNDERSTANDING ACTION

Yet another problem which plagues both the writer and the
reader of sociological work is the ambiguity of human
action. How can we be certain that such and such really
did mean what I say it meant? This difficulty is
heightened when the reader is presented with mere snippets
of data, abstracted from the context in which they occurred - a procedure which is clearly essential when data
are long and monographs are short. As we shall see, there
are special difficulties involved in interpreting the kind
of data considered here. For all of these reasons some
comment is needed on the solutions that I adopted.
    For some writers the difficulty of providing guaranteed
interpretation of any datum has led to their rejection of
all conventional sociological description. While it is
certainly true that all hitherto existing sociologies have
failed to provide any sure method for overcoming the ambiguities of meaning in social interaction, it would be
absurd to argue that such inquiry was thereby invalid. (3)
The relevant arguments could and unfortunately do fill
many volumes. Two brief points may be made here.
    First, although misunderstanding is commonplace in
daily life, it is clear that most action is premised upon
the assumption that a correct interpretation of it is both
possible and likely, at least where the participants are
familiar with the situation. Indeed, action is constructed very precisely so that it can be correctly in-
terpreted by the competent insider. (4) Thus for the
outsider who wishes to understand what is going on, the
principal method of arriving at this is to try to become
competent, to immerse oneself as fully as possible in the
situation; which is, of course, the procedure adopted in
this study.
    One further source of help is also available. Since
misunderstanding is still a common occurrence, whatever
the participants' competence, they are obliged to take the
possibility of failure continually into account. Indeed,
in responding to one another we openly display that we
have understood the previous speakers' meaning in order to
establish our reply as a relevant one. (5) Thus the

students of interaction can be guided in their reading of
these matters, not just by their familiarity with the
scene but by the readings displayed by the participants.
Neither procedure guarantees an objective interpretation,
but the use of both may help to generate a substantial
measure of confidence in the analysis.

So far, so good. It must be noted, however, that the
extent and manner in which meanings and understandings are
displayed varies greatly, and this may add considerably to
the difficulty of the analysts' task. In any interaction
a large number of different things are conveyed and some
are much more liable to misinterpretation than others.
The main reason for this is simple: participants typically differ in the extent to which they have shared
membership in the various social worlds under discussion.

To take the example of doctor-patient consultations:
it is notorious that certain messages are extremely difficult to convey. Doctors, for instance, often experience
great difficulty in understanding the world in which their
patients live and may operate with a set of stereotypes
quite inappropriate to that world (e.g., see Macintyre,
1977).

By contrast there are other matters in which both
doctors and patients typically share some competence and
about which they can communicate with facility. Such
would seem to be the case with the matters under consideration here. That is, with the exception of some of the
Puerto Rican patients in the American hospitals, all the
adult participants in these medical consultations demonstrated considerable awareness of the rules of the ceremonial order of clinics. (6)

This shared competence can present considerable analytical difficulties, greater perhaps than those found
where misunderstanding is common. For where both parties
are insiders, communication as to the nature of the world
they share is typically indirect and allusive and, although meanings and understandings are certainly displayed, this is normally done in the most delicate of
fashions. In such cases rules are spelt out only in
special circumstances, as when, for example, they have
been broken or when outsiders are present. Since this is
done only to the deviant or the ignorant, to name a rule
is to name a person and must necessarily be done with discretion if one is not to formulate oneself as incompetent
or offensive.

In consequence, although I have quoted several examples
in which rules were actually spelt out, these occurred but
a mere handful of times. Since rules were openly formulated only in special circumstances, such occasions cannot

be cited as direct evidence of normal rule use but are
instead something different: acts of teaching, warning
or attempted mitigation.

This general absence of relevant formulations in the
interaction means that we are faced with a paradox.
Interviewing generates spoken or written statements of
rules, either made by or agreed with by the respondents.
These can be openly displayed and sometimes even counted
by the researcher. However, there is no way of knowing
how these rules relate to and are used in actual behaviour. By contrast, the observation and recording of
relatively trouble-free interaction provides extremely
rich data on 'what happens', but few if any occasions on
which we may actually see or hear the rules being
followed.

Quite what the rules are is therefore unclear at first.
This difficulty is compounded by two further features.
For a start, the same rule may be embodied in a great
variety of very different behaviour according to circumstance. I have already noted how no rule contains within
it the further set of criteria for its application on particular occasions. Observation certainly permits the researcher to gather extensive data on the differing ways in
which the same rule may be applied. But since rules are
not normally formulated during action, still less their
rules of use, seeing the same rule across a wide range of
encounters presents considerable difficulties, as does the
display of that rule in its various natural habitats so
that others may see it too.

The other difficulty is this. Following a rule concerns the omission of certain behaviour as much as the
commission of other behaviour. Here not even the acts,
let alone the rules, are directly audible or visible.
Absences are as important as presences; but to notice
that the dog did not bark in the night is often a most
difficult task and one that is even harder to prove unless
one can display all of one's data.

UNDERSTANDING AND FORMULATING RULES

There are certain solutions to the problems of finding and
displaying tacit social rules with the use of observational data. These procedures were used in the analysis of
the material discussed here and inform the logic, such as
it is, of its presentation. Apart from the special case
that I have already cited where rules were already spelt
out, six types of data have been presented to warrant the
finding of a particular rule, though, given the limi-

tations of time, space and enthusiasm, not all six have
been listed for every rule.

First, I have given examples of typical and entirely
routine uses. I hope this gives the reader some flavour
of standard usage but it does not, as we have seen,
necessarily display that this was indeed the rule being
followed in the behaviour cited. Nor does such quotation
adequately establish just what was omitted. For these
purposes a second type of example is necessary. Although
this book is principally concerned with the nature of the
bureaucratic format in medical consultations, the rather
different behaviour found in the other formats, when contrasted with that found within the bureaucratic type,
gives a much clearer indication of the basic rules within
the latter.

This contrast may illuminate just what is involved by
the rules of the bureaucratic format, but it leaves untouched the problem of demonstrating the range of these
rules and their universal application within this range.
The scope of the rules has been shown first by a consideration of their outer edges, the limiting cases in which
they do not apply. These form a third type of data. One
analytical strategy in these cases is to show that, although these are counter-examples, they are produced by
very special circumstances and occur only within these.

To demonstrate that the rule was applied consistently,
apart from these special circumstances, has required a
fourth kind of data. This may be divided into two types.
First, one needs a selection of examples which display a
cross-section of the kinds of occasion on which the rule
is necessary. Second and more importantly, one requires
a detailed consideration of those situations which would
seem to threaten the applicability of the rule. In other
words, to establish a rule's universality one needs to
examine those occasions on which it is most seriously
tested. For example, in analysing the rule that the
doctor is always the expert, the crucial test becomes
what happens when the parents do in fact possess medical
knowledge.

A fifth type of data has concerned the extent to which
the rule varies systematically in use. So far I have considered only the problems of finding and displaying the
most general form of a rule. But rules vary in their
manner of use according to circumstances, and this too
must be demonstrated. For example, all parents were
treated as if they were moral, loving, intelligent and
honest; but as regards their competence vis-à-vis the
child there were important differences. Mothers' competence was totally assumed; that of fathers was openly
questioned.

A final and sixth type of data has come from the discussion of these rules in interviews with doctors. Such
data present considerable problems for analysis if the researcher has no other; but, taken together with the other
data sources that have been outlined, they act as both a
check and a useful guide.

THE GENERATION AND TESTING OF HYPOTHESES

A brief comment is necessary about the way in which the
ideas in this study were produced and tested. There are
various systematic methods for analysing qualitative data,
and the procedure used here was a mixture of that which
Glaser (1964) has termed the 'constant comparative method
of qualitative analysis' and the method of 'analytic
induction' as described by Robinson (1951), Cressey (1971)
and Bloor (1976b). Both are alternatives to the
hypothetico-deductive or 'big bang' mode of analysis that
is normally used with pre-coded data. In this latter mode
one systematically deduces a set of hypotheses from a body
of theory and attempts to falsify them at one go. By contrast, analytic induction attempts to relate the process
of generating propositions more closely to the data.
Explanations are tested out all the time, trying them on
one case to see if they fit, then moving on to another,
and so on. Where the proposition does not cover the particular case, it may be reformulated or else the phenomenon redefined until a universal relationship is established which fits all the cases.
     For its successful use the method of analytic induction
requires a precise formulation of at least part of the
problem. However, the research described here had
initially no one focus but several overlapping ones. To
begin with I had no intention of studying the doctor-
patient role-relationship since I held 'role' to be an
old-fashioned and exploded concept. It was only at a late
stage in the project and as a result of writing on various
other themes that I became convinced that there were clear
structures here. Making up one's mind as late as this has
important disadvantages. If I had discovered this earlier
on I could have designed the study far more systematically
to test my propositions. Since I did not, I was faced
with a dilemma. On the one hand, I needed a method that
would enable the generation of a coherent set of ideas but
that would also, at least initially, leave matters
somewhat open and offer scope for modification. On the
other hand, once I had a series of propositions, I required a method that would enable me to test them in some
relatively adequate form.

In consequence, I began the analysis with a method that had a strong resemblance to the 'constant comparative method' proposed by Glaser. He argues that

... in contrast to analytic induction the method is concerned with generating and plausibly suggesting (not provisionally testing) many properties and hypotheses about a *general* phenomenon (Glaser, 1964, p.438).

As its name implies, this method consists of comparing each datum with a given selection of categories and seeing whether or not it fits. Once one has coded for a category several times and developed a more sophisticated version of it, one then codes only if the datum that is being examined points to a new aspect of the category. The only exception to this are categories of great theoretical interest but of which there are very few examples. If the datum fits under none of them, then the categories are modified or an entirely new one produced. The aim is to bring whatever initial ideas one has systematically to the data, and in the process of this to see what new ideas can be generated. Once all the data have been examined, the material relating to each is systematically scrutinized and further sub-divisions or re-groupings made, as items are found to differ or cluster together.

In my use of this method I made one important modification. This process of hypothesis generation was carried out on only one half of the data, with most of the material from the American hospital and most of that from the Scottish neurological clinic being excluded. Having completed the initial analysis of the first half of the data, I then re-organized my basic categories according to my current ideas, re-analysed the coded data and wrote a first, though only partial, draft. This provided me with a systematic set of propositions which I was then able to test by analysing the further half of my data. Where these did not fit the argument was amended. This latter step rendered my analysis, in this instance, more akin to the method of analytic induction.

Notes

CHAPTER 1 INTRODUCTION

1   For a definition of the ritual order see Goffman
    (1975a). As he points out, we seem to lack a word
    which captures the full meaning of this order.
    'Ritual' is not quite right because it does not convey
    the fact that matters of considerable substantive
    import are involved. None of the alternatives in
    sociological use are any better: 'ceremony', 'po-
    liteness', 'expressive' - all fail in this respect.
    Our secularized culture makes such a sharp division
    between the practical world and that of ceremony that
    we have no terms left with which to grasp the intense-
    ly moral and ritual nature of the way in which we
    frame our practical concerns.
2   This distinction cannot be pushed too far as there are
    also resemblances between the forms of different kinds
    of service relationship (Wenglinsky, 1973; Strong,
    1977a).
3   For a more extended critique of Parsons's model see
    Bloor and Horobin (1975), and Strong and Davis (1977).
4   This model is considered in more detail in chapter 8.
    Perhaps the best introduction to it is contained in
    Goffman (1961).
5   A more systematic if far less detailed comparison of
    these formats is contained in Strong and Davis (1977).
    Note also that the analysis of Goffman presented in
    this article is somewhat different from that given in
    this book. This change is due principally to my
    reading the paper by Gonos (1977) on Goffman.
6   This article is concerned solely with the use of the
    game format in therapists' work with children. How-
    ever, the same mode was also used by doctors in the
    developmental assessment of young children. Indeed,

it would seem to be a standard format available to any adult in our culture for use with the very young.

7 This is not entirely fair to Goffman, since one of his central themes has been the micropolitics of encounters; that is, how people use frames to suit their own particular ends (Goffman, 1970, 1971a). Indeed, for many readers Goffman presents too cynical a view of interaction. His very concern with the relationship of individuals to frames leads him to treat frames themselves as given, a tendency that is reinforced by his failure to consider either the range of frames in use within any one activity-system, or their historical origins, or their current uses. These matters are discussed more fully in chapter 8.

8 See Bittner's (1965) formulation of how official plans are used in this fashion in organizations.

9 The attempt to make one set of standards apply to each and every action and encounter is, of course, the definition of radicalism. As Bittner (1963) has shown, such attempts necessarily fail and indeed those radical movements that survive do so only by creating elaborate procedures for enabling their members to ignore those large areas of reality that do not fit their creed.

CHAPTER 2   MEDICAL SYSTEMS AND SETTINGS

1 For most practical purposes there is no difference between the NHS in Scotland and the NHS in England and Wales. For other general sociological comparisons between the British and American systems, see Freidson (1970a) and Mechanic (1971). For a more personal account of the NHS see Roth (1977), as well as a view by an American doctor (Fisher, 1974). All these comparisons are by American authors.

2 It should be noted that the Scottish city was famed for the degree to which such services were planned, centralized and to some extent imposed upon the population. Although these features are characteristic of the British health services as a whole when compared with American health services, the Scottish city displayed them to an unusual degree.

3 Interestingly, there was one medical institution in the Scottish city that did promote itself somewhat in the American fashion. This was a hospital for the long-term care of severely retarded children. These institutions have been starved of public funds, and such promotion is one way of redeeming the balance.

An assessment and nursery centre for handicapped
children which opened at the end of the study also
began to promote itself along the same lines.

4 One must not over-emphasize the extent to which
records were linked. The GP and hospital record
systems were not themselves linked, nor were the local
authority records linked to the hospital, or vice
versa.

5 Given the importance of medical conditions as a source
of variation in the nature of consultations, it would
be useful to quantify these. However, although large
numbers of different kinds of condition were seen in
the course of the research, to give precise figures
here would be merely guesswork. This would make sense
only if it were based on a detailed analysis of the
patient records; and although this was attempted for
a selection of 60 cases for the Scottish neurological
clinic it proved immensely problematic. The three
researchers spent a month each on this task, and to
have studied them all would have been impossible.
Moreover, one is not comparing like with like. The
term 'diagnosis' covers very different types of
entity. 'Headaches' for example are symptoms, while
others such as 'fall' are assertions about cause, and
yet others, such as 'spina bifida', are simply descriptions (Blaxter, 1978). Finally, the process of
diagnosis is a phenomenon of varying method and
accuracy. Different doctors may produce different
diagnoses, and any one diagnosis may have a differing
degree of certainty from case to case and consultation
to consultation.

CHAPTER 3   NATURAL PARENTHOOD

1 Macintyre (1976) has commented on a rather similar
reification of character in medical work with pregnant
women, though two important differences from this
should be noted. Reification in children's clinics
was a matter of surface ceremony; it did not necessarily reflect what staff actually thought of mothers.
The same character was ascribed to mothers whatever
their marital or other status; whereas, as Macintyre
shows, 'maternal instincts' were presumed to occur
only in married women while the single but pregnant
woman 'naturally' wished to be rid of her child.

2 For an analysis of the reconstitution of character,
see Garfinkel (1956b). Note also that face-work is
not tied to the preservation of the good, nor is

character-work to the denunciation of the bad. Where
a player is cast as a villain, then face-work may be
essential to preserve this image of evil; conversely,
even the worst sinners may be redeemed.

3 The charity mode has the least empirical foundation of
any format considered in this study. Although it is
based on the work of only one doctor and there are
likely to be some idiosyncratic elements within this
particular usage, there is some evidence from other
studies that its central feature - explicit moral investigation - can be found in a rather similar form
elsewhere. Recent studies of British casualty departments have described the open denunciation of
certain disreputable cases such as repeat suicide
attempts and drunks (Jeffreys, 1974; Gibson, 1977);
and Byrne and Long (1976, pp.57-8) give a detailed
illustration of the lengths to which character-work
may go in general practice - if very rarely. Thus,
although such behaviour seems most unusual, it clearly
does exist in places. There was also a hint in the
Scottish hospital that such scenes had not been
unknown in the past. Here, for instance, are a
doctor's comments to his students after seeing a case
of severe nappy rash and asking the mother to come in
to the mother and baby unit:

> Dr G: She doesn't seem very well cared for, but
> then it is her first baby.

He says that the nurses will teach her how to look
after a baby properly.

> Dr G: They do it much better than in the old days.
> The old nurses were very dictatorial. They
> snatched babies away from mothers as soon as
> they came in if they suspected they weren't
> well looked after. Now they teach them much
> more surreptitiously ... (pause) ... I hope
> ... (laughter).

4 This division is similar to that found in other
studies of judgmental work (Emerson, 1969; Macintyre,
1977).

5 Of the 18 occasions on which fathers alone brought the
child, 11 consultations took place in the Scottish
neurological clinic; one in the Scottish general
medical clinic; 4 in the Scottish occupational therapy department, in so far as those can be called
consultations; and on two occasions in the American

    clinics. Since one father attended several times and in two different settings the total number of fathers seen on their own was 13.

6 One other point should be noted about the treatment that fathers received when present with their spouses. Although I have argued that they had a subordinate position in clinics, it was more common for wives to check their remarks with their partner than for husbands to do this. Many wives looked towards their husbands for their assent; their husbands only rarely reciprocated when they themselves spoke. This, coupled with the fact that it was fathers who often asked the more awkward questions – a point which I shall raise later, suggests that although mothers were given some priority in medical consultations, their authority as regards their children was not as absolute as might be gathered just from this account.

CHAPTER 4   COLLEGIAL AUTHORITY

1 Since no check was made on patient records, this analysis is based only on the cases in which I was informed that the cases were private.

2 'From the point of view of the authority, the important issue about any act becomes, not whether it is performed in accordance with a particular rule, but whether it is performed in accordance with the rule establishing authority itself' (Werthmann, 1969, p.620).

3 I have not considered the fourth case here, since it was so complex. Even though the dispute was left unresolved, its main elements did seem to conform to the general picture I have drawn in this chapter. What appears to have happened is that the mother, who was extremely dubious about the usefulness of treatment offered by the doctor, was afraid to say so directly but instead gave a whole series of seemingly absurd excuses for not being able to fix a definite time for the next appointment, each of which provoked the doctor into yet more detailed investigation of these reasons. As the doctor's grumpiness increased so did the mother's, until she gave an angry denunciation of the treatment her child had had at the clinic. Both parties then cooled down; but the mother left without having fixed a definite time for a new appointment and did not in fact return.

4 It could, however, be argued that extreme non-verbal dissent is partly designed to enforce an investigation

by the superior party, thus drawing some of the sting
from a subordinate's challenge by making it a requested item. (This may well have been part of the
reasoning behind the bizarre excuses given by the
mother described in note 3, above). Perhaps it is
better to leave intentions out of this altogether
and merely state that such behaviour is a typical
response by the weak, and that, whatever its motivation on any particular occasion, it can produce
the above effects.

5 These 20 cases were seen in 7 different settings, 5 in
Scotland and 2 in America, and involved 10 different
staff members, all but one a doctor. Since no check
was made on patient records this total is based on
what was mentioned in clinics. It may well have some
accuracy, for staff routinely inquired about parents'
occupations for the records, while a visit from a
parent with medical connections was a matter for
warning by nurses and general comment between staff.
They were well aware of the threat posed by such
parents. Note also that there was no difference
between the private and bureaucratic formats in
respect of the problems that such parents presented
or the treatment they received. Thus I have included,
within this total of 20 cases, 2 private patients from
the American hospital.

6 This does not mean that these parents presented no
threat to staff's authority, merely that they obeyed
the surface ceremony. Beneath that ceremony, some of
these parents in fact mounted very severe challenges
(see chapter 8).

CHAPTER 5 A JOINT VENTURE

1 Goffman (1971a) contains a very detailed treatment of
a whole range of 'illegitimate' motives and interests
that the providers of services may have, and of the
ways in which these are concealed. Doctors are not
alone in their problems.
2 A television series, 'Dr Finlay's Casebook', which
concerned general practice in the Scottish Highlands
in the 1920s.

CHAPTER 6 MEDICAL CONTROL

1 The past neglect in medical sociology of the influence
of patients upon medical consultations has led in

recompense to some exaggeration of that influence.
The interactionist tradition is famous for demonstrating that the lower orders in organizations have
more power than they have been conventionally
ascribed. It is equally famous, or perhaps notorious,
for the neglect of the way in which those normally
thought to be powerful do in fact exercise their
control. The irony which is one of the main strengths
of the tradition is always in danger of degenerating
into whimsy.

2   There is one important exception to this. Parents did
not attempt any direct manipulation of the audience,
but they did have one powerful source of indirect
manipulation. There seemed to be a general rule that
absolutely all adults, no matter what the situation,
were obliged to smile and wonder at a young child if
called upon to do so by mothers. Those parents of
handicapped children who resisted the doctors' diagnosis commonly appealed to this rule to divert the
conversation on to other matters. By calling for
shared wonderment they seemed to hope that others
would be forced to agree that their child was normal
(see Davis and Strong, 1976b).

3   Heath (1978) gives a detailed analysis of the cen-
trality of records to general practice consultation
and the way doctors are able to conjure elaborate
performances out of just a few fragments of notes.

4   Doctors could also use official form-filling to indicate that nothing very serious was at issue. The
questions on the developmental assessment forms in the
local authority clinics were not normally differentiated from each other. All were asked with the same
light and routine air, even though some doctors asked
for more precision than others. It should also be
noted that some of the junior American doctors who did
the work-up, which was also a highly standardized
affair, did so in a heavily bureaucratic manner as if
to display their subordinate status. They were
filling in a form for the Chief and not for themselves.

5   One of the parents seen at the developmental clinic in
the American hospital was however reported to have
made notes on a previous visit. He had apparently
already visited numerous hospitals across the United
States in an attempt to have his son defined as normal
rather than retarded. The staff suspected that the
notes were to aid him in legal action against the
hospital; they turned out to be notes on the test
procedures, made so that he could coach his son for
the next visit.

6 For an analysis of small talk and the concepts of pre-
and post-activity talk see Turner (1972).

7 In this study I have not attempted to analyse systematically the specific routines used by individual
doctors. That such routines existed was obvious, for
note-taking became far more rapid and accurate once a
doctor's particular style had been 'learnt'. The best
evidence for the distinct but highly routinized nature
of diagnostic practice is Bloor's (1976a, 1976b)
detailed study of adeno-tonsillectomy decision-making
by eleven ENT surgeons. Note also that although the
routinization of practice was more immediately obvious
when staff worked to an official form, this should not
be taken to mean that such forms imposed a common set
of routines on all who used them. Different doctors
used the form in different ways. The crucial point
is that individually those ways were heavily routinized.

8 The only exception to this rule was the developmental
clinic in the American hospital, where the doctors
worked together with a social worker. The latter
watched the child being assessed through a one-way
screen, and afterwards the two staff members went into
emotional matters with parents. Although several assessment sessions were observed, the researchers were
excluded from the later proceedings. The clinic was
seen as a special venture by the hospital and saw very
few patients compared with the Scottish neurological
clinic. The introduction of strong emotions into
medical work seems likely to represent a major break
with the bureaucratic format.

9 This analysis is based solely on cases observed in the
Scottish clinics, since the only American children
seen with serious conditions who had attended the
hospital over a long period were seen in the amphitheatre clinic. This setting, as will be seen in the
next chapter, was not typical of other clinics within
the hospital. Such children were certainly patients
of these latter clinics, but unfortunately none were
observed in the brief American visit.

CHAPTER 7 EASE AND TENSION IN THE ALLIANCE

1 Although staff shared, at least at this basic level,
a common set of categories for classifying parents, I
do not mean to suggest that there was any necessary
agreement about who was and who was not dim, sensible,
bright, and so on. Just as they differed over their

right to moralize, so too different staff applied
these categories in different ways, something which
on a few, rare occasions led to fierce internal
disputes.

2 This rule did not apply with such force in the more
regular and less formal therapy sessions. In consequence, therapists felt themselves better able to
judge the normal level of care which children received.

3 The amphitheatre clinic gave even greater prominence
to the clinical format than the Scottish clinic.
Indeed, where the parents could not speak competent
English or where a child was unaccompanied by parents,
the clinical format was almost totally dominant, a
fact which resulted in tears in some younger children
and great offence in adolescents.

4 The difficulties that such problems caused for the
overall promise of medicine are similar to those that
they also cause for religious faith. Religion, like
medicine, both distinguishes between a natural and a
social world and yet invests the natural world with
moral meaning. Fatal or handicapping conditions have
thus always presented religions with difficulties in
accounting for their existence. Voysey (1975) discusses some of the 'theodicies', or justifications of
the existence of God in the face of evil, that have
been developed to explain handicap. Modern medical
theodicy rests on the promise that disease will be
overcome by scientific research and manipulation – a
programme which has recently come in for considerable
criticism. Many have challenged humankind's right and
ability to master 'nature' in this way. The most
famous critique of medical aspirations is that of
Illich (1975), whose own theodicy is fundamentally
religious: pain and suffering are not things to be
overcome but to be accepted as teaching us about life.

5 Davis and Strong (1976b) contains a more detailed
analysis of the conditions for ease in such circumstances.

6 These 26 consultations took place in 6 different
settings and involved 9 doctors; no foster-mother was
seen in a therapy department. Of the 17 foster-
mothers, three were seen in the general paediatric
clinics in the American hospital and at least one was
seen in each of the types of Scottish clinic, although
all the repeat cases were seen in the neurological
clinic.

7 There were, however, some similarities with the position that natural mothers found themselves in. A

foster-mother might well lose her job if a doctor complained, while she was often accompanied to the clinic
by a social worker from her employing agency. Her
professional competence was therefore on the line on
such occasions.

8 A total of 12 Scottish local-authority social workers
were seen in clinics. None accompanied a child by
themselves but most were present with foster-mothers,
unlike the 11 house-mothers who in all but one case
were a child's sole representative in a clinic.
Neither of these kinds of professional was observed in
the American consultations. It should be noted that
part of the praise which foster-mothers were so openly
given might well be due to the tensions between
doctors and social workers from outside agencies. To
compliment a foster-mother might be a subtle way of
putting down the social worker who, by implication,
knew less and was doing less good. Such battles were
normally fought indirectly, but some indication of the
major challenge which social workers represented may
be gained from the following excerpt, where the doctor
is attacked in a fashion never dared by any parent:

> SW: The parents adopting the child do have the
>   right to know its background.
> Dr I: Yes. (They briefly discuss another topic.)
> SW: So much depends on the medical side.
> Dr I: What do you mean?
> SW: Well, on this examination.
> Dr I: Well, I'll write and say that I think there
>   is a very small risk and no more and that
>   he's OK for adoption, with this proviso.
> SW: Well (significantly) There is a problem of
>   course.

The foster-mother left the room and the social worker
then repeated at length what she had said about their
duty to adopting parents and how they would have to
tell them everything about the child. The doctor
repeated his remarks. This did not seem to satisfy
the social worker, who repeated her arguments several
more times. Eventually she broke off with a sigh and
stood up to leave. But then she added:

> SW: We had a lot of trouble with that last child
>   we had from you.
> Dr I: Well, you didn't have it from me. You've
>   never had a child from me.
> SW: No ... (pause, then adding significantly) ...

> But it was from *here,* wasn't it? (Doctor looks
> blank and does not reply.) Ah, well, doctor,
> goodbye.
> Dr I: Goodbye.

CHAPTER 8 CONCLUSIONS AND GENERALIZATIONS

1 See in particular 'Fun in Games' (Goffman, 1961).
2 The originality and importance of this model is well
   brought out in Helmer (1970).
3 See 'Role Distance' (Goffman, 1961) and, in particular, his recent critique of the over-deterministic
   use of framing in conversational analysis (Goffman,
   1975b). Here Goffman argues that the whole concept of
   frame is no more than a useful fiction, a heuristic
   pretence that action is so determined when in fact it
   is not:

> Thus the whole framework of conversational con-
> straints - both system and ritual - can become
> something to honor, to invert, or to disregard, de-
> pending as the mood strikes. It's not that the lid
> can't be closed; there is no box (Goffman, 1975b,
> p.35).

4 Note that this is the only study in which Goffman
   systematically observed and recorded the workings of
   a particular activity-system. Yet, having done so,
   he concentrated not so much on the frame itself but
   on the ways in which members distanced themselves from
   it.
5 The two instances of this phenomenon were: first, the
   two knowledgeable parents who were granted a semi-
   collegial status; and second, all those occasions
   when teaching was carried out. It may be objected
   that this latter activity forms a quite separate
   system of its own. Although this is true, the clinical format which partly informed this activity represented an alternative mode which could have been used
   to frame the interaction with parents.
6 This passage is cited in the first chapter of this
   volume.
7 These metaphors are more fully developed in the work
   of Weinstein (1964,1966,1969), though he too is concerned only with the genesis of particular encounters
   and not with the generation of formats.
8 Once again it is slightly unfair to accuse Goffman of
   not being aware of the reification of formats. He

typically has most things covered in an aside or a
footnote somewhere:

> I can only suggest that he who would combat false
> consciousness and awaken people to their true
> interests has much to do, because the sleep is very
> deep. And I do not intend here to provide a
> lullaby but merely to sneak in and watch the way
> the people snore (Goffman, 1975a, p.12).

Nevertheless, one may legitimately argue that the political and historical aspect of formats is neglected
in Goffman's work and constitutes perhaps its major
omission (Annett and Collins, 1975). See also the
excellent political analysis of a format in Barth
(1966).

9 This analysis suggests that it is part of the human
   condition to move continually back and forth between
   reified and instrumental versions of social form. The
   belief that we can create a de-reified world is
   therefore as illusory as the closely-related search
   for guaranteed knowledge. Illusions can, however, be
   most important. The fact that we shall never arrive
   at the truth should not prevent us from seeking it out
   as best we can; our inability to construct a fully
   rational world need not deter us from trying.

10 A much fuller account of some of these properties is
   given in Davis and Strong (1976b).

11 For an excellent description of sustained childish
   defiance see Werthman (1969).

12 This seems to be borne out by a study of interaction
   in an outpatient clinic at an adult hospital in which
   I am currently engaged.

13 The direct financial interest in gaining extra trade
   that exists in a private practice system may weaken
   professional standards, for doctors may end up selling
   services that the client wants rather than those in
   which they themselves believe. Private clients can
   shop around until they find a doctor to certify that
   they have the disease they think they have, but in
   non-competitive systems people have to make do with
   the doctor's version. There was a distinct tendency
   for the American hospital to validate new diseases
   promoted by parental pressure-groups in a more whole-
   hearted fashion than their Scottish colleagues.
   Middle-class American parents could more readily
   choose whether their child had 'learning disability'
   or was 'autistic'. See also Freidson's (1970b, pp.
   91-3) distinction between client- and colleague-
   dependent practice.

14 Note that this analysis also explains the standard use of the bureaucratic format in the American hospital in all but private patients. The Welfare State has come rather later to the United States and is still far less developed. Nevertheless, since federal and state governments now intervene on a large scale in medicine, poor patients carry some political weight; for hospitals are heavily dependent on such funding, even the private foundations such as the one studied here.

15 A certain element of competition for patients does exist within the NHS: between highly specialized units which take referrals from all over the country, and also, if to a lesser extent, between general practitioners whose patients are free to register elsewhere (though this is not the easiest of moves) and who are paid directly in accordance with the number of patients on their register. This competitive pressure will therefore reinforce the pressure exerted by political power.

16 For a systematic treatment of the theories of Victorian burgesses on the rights of the individual and the role of the state see Poggi (1977).

17 By contrast, whereas any mother who attended the 'charity' clinic was an object of suspicion to the doctor, and simply to be there was to cast her character in doubt, the reverse assumption operated in the Scottish clinics. That parents, or at least most of them, were naturally loving and competent was not just for public consumption but was a deeply held belief. Their attendance at the hospital was prima facie evidence not of their incompetence but of their good character.

> Dr I: (to students) It's important to check on family circumstances because with a child showing delay you've always got to be on the look-out for emotional and social deprivation, but there's never been any hint of this here. *They've always kept appointments* [my emphasis] and so on, and Therapist F hasn't mentioned it, and this is one of the things she's on the look-out for.

18 These remarks should not be taken to mean that Soviet doctors and patients are normally subject to heavy political constraints. The typical doctor-patient relationship would seem to be of a heavily bourgeois kind. Freidson (1970a) ascribes this to the independent power which experts attain. I would see it

also as a product of working-class power. Its establishment in a Communist state has exactly the same
functions as it does in a capitalist state: it le-
gitimates the government and helps to buy off the op-
position. For both kinds of society are of the distinctly modern type in which, whether or not there are
genuine elections, there is nevertheless a mass participation in politics - what Barraclough (1967) calls
the *party-state* or what Bauman (1976), following
Bendix, calls *plebiscitarianism*.

19 See Scheff (1968) for an instructive analysis of the
way a psychiatrist can totally transform a presenting
problem. Such games may be fun to play and even
helpful at times. Whether they should interfere with
the business of ordinary doctoring is another matter.

20 Modern psychotherapy has of course a distinctly
bourgeois flavour, with its emphasis on 'non-
directive' techniques and its goal of 'self-
realization'. Nevertheless, while still connected
with the doctrine of individualism, such beliefs seem
highly destructive of its core - and more readily compatible with a collectivist vision of the world. It
can be argued that techniques like encounter groups
are devices by which investigative character-work may
be carried out while leaving the therapists' hands
clean - one simply gets the patients to do character-
work on each other. It is precisely because of its
bourgeois trimmings that psychotherapy is so much more
saleable a commodity than Samuel Butler's vision of a
fully social version of medicine. It should also be
noted that in some full-blown psychotherapeutic
doctrines even diseases like cancer are transformed
into personal rather than bodily malignancies. For a
fervent modern statement of the bourgeois position on
the naturalness of illness see Sontag (1978).

21 The trends are contradictory here. The United States
has a far more self-obsessed culture than that of
Britain, and is the principal home of psychotherapy.
The increasingly popular 'family medicine' (Janeway,
1974) (a medical training which is half organic medicine and half psychiatry) has no equivalent in British
medical schools, despite the popularity of Balint in
some departments of general practice. On the other
hand, the relative lack of choice between practitioners under the NHS means that it would be less easy for
the British patient to escape if a more social version
of medicine was introduced. An instructive account of
how the system can already operate, with a child
patient deemed to need psychiatric treatment by

doctors but not by parents, can be found in Roth (1977).

22   The special assessment and treatment unit for handicapped children which opened at the end of this study
seems to have provided a more personal service than
was previously available in outpatient clinics. At
any rate, parents who had experience of both services
drew a sharp distinction between them (Gibson, 1977).

23   Of course there may be some occasions when doctors too
believe that parents were at least partly responsible.
Even here however it is normally kinder to place these
things firmly in a natural frame.

CHAPTER 9   A METHODOLOGICAL APPENDIX

1   My stress here is upon capacities, not upon actual
counting practices, for clearly there may be some
things which people could count if they so chose but
which only social scientists have any interest in.
Moreover, there are some tribes where arithmetic is
so under-developed that the precise counting of
anything stops at a handful.

2   See the marvellous critique of 'quantophrenia' and the
rise of the accountants in social science in Sorokin
(1956).

3   Some authors have been so disturbed by the failure to
generate foolproof interpretive methods that they have
abandoned all interest in conventional subject-matters
and concentrated solely on analysing the methods that
are used in everyday life to this end; their hope
being that here at least some certainty is to be
found. The more optimistic of them have an essentially Cartesian strategy. They have deliberately sus-
pended belief in all the things that sociologists
normally claim to know, hoping that if some small
area of life can be found about which knowledge can
be truly guaranteed, then a proper sociology might
eventually be constructed on this firm basis. While
this quest for certainty has produced some brilliant
studies of lay methodology and the structuring of
talk, the larger programme is surely a delusion and
is likely, for all its rigour, to go the way of the
many previous attempts to find epistemological
bedrock. The best we can hope for in this world, even
if we study practical reasoning, is a plausible story.

4   Paradoxically, if competent insiders could not normally grasp the meaning of events, deceit would prove a
most difficult matter. Its ready accomplishment

depends on others both continuing to operate with the
premise that things are as they seem and possessing
the skills to interpret things in the normal fashion.
Sudnow (1972) gives a nice example of this in his
paper on glancing. As he shows, it is a central
property of social scenes that they can be understood
at a glance, at least by those familiar with them.
They are indeed skilfully constructed in order that
insiders can so read them, and dissimulation merely
uses the same procedures to different ends.

5 See Goffman (1975b, pp.13-15) for an elaboration of
this point. Some may object that, although this is
true, one cannot have any proper confidence in the
readings one makes until the procedures by which
meaning and understanding are displayed have been
fully analysed and are available to the sociological
researcher. The weakness in this argument is that
there are no good grounds for restricting it to sociologists; and applied generally it becomes ridicu-
lous. If this were in fact the case, no one could
become competent in any social sphere without formal
instruction in ethnomethodology. If the laity can
acquire a working competence in these matters, one
sufficient for their purposes, I see no reason why
constructive sociologists cannot do the same.

6 Quite why this is so is beyond the scope of this monograph. It is not surprising that doctors and therapists should have this facility, since this is their
daily task, but parents' ability here poses more of a
problem. The competence shown by the great majority
of parents in this study would seem to derive from
three main sources. First, certain of the rules
relate to identities which are in standard use in our
culture, e.g., our images of mothers, fathers and
childhood. Second, as I suggest in chapter 8, it
seems likely that the bureaucratic role format is,
with minor modifications, in standard use across large
areas of medical practice. Most parents will
therefore have had considerable experience of the
form. Finally, it is also likely that the bureaucratic format found in medical consultations has a
good deal in common with those used in many other
types of service relationship, though so far no
detailed comparison has been made between these.
(But see Bigus, 1972; Wenglinsky, 1973.)

Bibliography

ANNETT, J. and COLLINS, R. (1975), A Short History of
Deference and Demeanour, in R.Collins, 'Conflict
Sociology', Academic Press, New York.
ATKINSON, P. (1976), 'The Clinical Experience', Edinburgh,
unpublished Ph.D.
BALINT, E. and NORELL, J.S. (1973), 'Six Minutes for the
Patient', Tavistock, London.
BALINT, M. (1957), 'The Doctor, His Patient and the
Illness', Pitman Medical, London.
BARRACLOUGH, G. (1967), 'An Introduction to Contemporary
History', Penguin Books, Harmondsworth, Middlesex.
BARTH, F. (1966), 'Models of Social Organization', Royal
Anthropological Institute, London, Occasional Paper No.23.
BAUMAN, Z. (1976), 'Socialism: The Active Utopia', Allen
& Unwin, London.
BECKER, H. (1969a), Social Observation and Case Studies,
in his 'Sociological Work', Aldine, Chicago.
BECKER, H. (1969b), Fieldwork Evidence, in his 'Socio-
logical Work', Aldine, Chicago.
BENNETT, A.E. (1976), 'Communication Between Doctors and
Patients', Oxford University Press, Oxford.
BIGUS, O. (1972), The Milkman and His Customer: A
Cultivated Relationship, 'Urban Life and Culture', 1, pp.
131-65.
BITTNER, E. (1963), Radicalism and the Organization of
Radical Movements, 'American Sociological Review',
XXVIII, pp.928-40.
BITTNER, E. (1965), The Concept of Organization, 'Social
Research', 32, pp.239-55.
BLAXTER, M. (1978), Diagnosis as Category and Process, the
Case of Alcoholism, 'Social Science and Medicine', 12, 1A,
pp.9-18.
BLOOR, M. (1976a), 'Decision-Making in ENT Outpatient
Clinics and Variations in the Hospitalization of Children

for Adeno-Tonsillectomy', unpublished Ph.D. thesis,
Aberdeen University.
BLOOR, M. (1976b), Bishop Berkeley and the Adeno-
Tonsillectomy Enigma, 'Sociology', 10, 1, pp.43-61.
BLOOR, M. and HOROBIN, G. (1975), Conflict and Conflict
Resolutions in Doctor-Patient Interactions, in C.Cox and
A.Mead (eds), 'A Sociology of Medical Practice', Collier-
Macmillan, London.
BLUM, A. (1970), The Sociology of Mental Illness, in
J.Douglas (ed.), 'Deviance and Respectability: The Social
Construction of Moral Meanings', Basic Books, New York,
pp.36-60.
BRADLEY, I. (1976), 'The Call to Seriousness: The Evan-
gelical Impact on the Victorians', Jonathan Cape, London.
BUTLER, S. (1977), 'Erewhon'. Cited in R.Illsley et al.,
Everybody's Business? Concepts of Health and Illness,
p.13, in 'Health and Health Policy: Priorities for
Research', SSRC (UK).
BYRNE, P.S. and LONG, B.E.L. (1976), 'Doctors Talking to
Patients', HMSO, London.
CICOUREL, A. (1964), 'Method and Measurement in Soci-
ology', Free Press, New York.
CRESSEY, D. (1971), 'Other People's Money: A Study in the
Social Psychology of Embezzlement', Wadsworth, Belmont,
California.
DAVIS, A.G. (1978), 'Children and Medical Work', draft MS.
DAVIS, A.G. and STRONG, P.M. (1976a), The Management of a
Therapeutic Encounter, in M.Wadsworth and D.Robinson
(eds), 'Studies in Everyday Medical Life', Martin
Robertson, London, pp.123-37.
DAVIS, A.G. and STRONG, P.M. (1976b); Aren't Children
Wonderful? - A Study of the Allocation of Identity in
Developmental Assessment, in M.Stacey (ed.), 'The Soci-
ology of the National Health Service', Sociological Review
Monograph No.22, pp.156-75.
DAVIS, F. (1963), 'Passage Through Crisis: Polio Victims
and Their Families', Bobbs-Merrill, Indianapolis.
DINGWALL, R.W.J., Collectivism, Regionalism and Feminism:
Health Visiting and British Social Policy 1850-1975,
'Journal of Social Policy', 6, 1977, p.291.
DOUGLAS, J.D. (1971), introduction to 'Understanding
Everyday Life', ed. Douglas, J.D., Routledge & Kegan Paul,
London, pp.3-44.
EMERSON, R. (1969), 'Judging Delinquents', Aldine,
Chicago.
FINGARETTE, H. (1969), 'Self-Deception', Routledge & Kegan
Paul, London.
FISHER, R.L. (1974), A Connecticut Yankee in Great
Britain: Report of a Travelling Fellowship, 'Hartford
Hospital Bulletin', 29, 1, pp.349-54.

FLETCHER, C.M. (1973), 'Communication in Medicine', Nuffield Provincial Hospitals Trust, London.

FREIDSON, E. (1961), 'Patients' Views of Medical Practice', Russell Sage, New York.

FREIDSON, E. (1970a), 'Profession of Medicine', Dodd, Mead, New York.

FREIDSON, E. (1970b), 'Professional Dominance', Atherton, New York.

GARFINKEL, H. (1956a), Some Sociological Concepts and Methods for Psychiatrists, 'Psychiatric Research Reports', 6, pp.181-95.

GARFINKEL, H. (1956b), Conditions of Successful Degradation Ceremonies, 'American Journal of Sociology', 61, pp.420-4.

GIBSON, H. (1977), Rules, Routines and Records: The Work of an Accident and Emergency Department, unpublished Ph.D. thesis, Aberdeen University.

GLASER, B. (1964), The Constant Comparative Method of Qualitative Analysis, 'Social Problems', 12, pp.436-45.

GOFFMAN, E. (1961), 'Encounters', Bobbs-Merrill, Indianapolis.

GOFFMAN, E. (1963), 'Behaviour in Public Places', Free Press, New York.

GOFFMAN, E. (1968a), 'Asylums', Penguin, Harmondsworth, Middlesex.

GOFFMAN, E. (1968b), 'Stigma: Notes on the Management of Spoiled Identity', Penguin, Harmondsworth, Middlesex.

GOFFMAN, E. (1970), 'Strategic Interaction', Basil Blackwell, Oxford.

GOFFMAN, E. (1971a), 'The Presentation of Self in Everyday Life', Penguin, Harmondsworth, Middlesex.

GOFFMAN, E. (1971b), 'Relations in Public', Penguin, Harmondsworth, Middlesex.

GOFFMAN, E. (1972), 'Interaction Ritual', Penguin, Harmondsworth, Middlesex.

GOFFMAN, E. (1975a), 'Frame Analysis', Penguin, Harmondsworth, Middlesex.

GOFFMAN, E. (1975b), Replies and Responses, 'Working Papers and Pre-publications', Centro Internazionale di Semiotica e di Linguistica, Urbino, pp.1-42,46-7.

GONOS, G. (1977), 'Situation' versus 'Frame': the 'Interactionist' and the 'Structuralist' Analyses of Everyday Life, 'American Sociological Review', 42, pp. 854-67.

HEATH, C. (1978), Some Interactional Features of Doctor-Patient Consultations: The Social Organization of Medical Record Cards and Non-Spoken Activity Episodes, unpublished Ph.D. thesis, Manchester University.

HELMER, J. (1970), The Face of the Man Without Qualities, 'Social Research', 37, pp.547-79.

HILLIARD, R., RAYNER, G. and SILVERMAN, D. (1977), The 'Patient-Centred' Model in a Hospital Setting: A Pilot Study of a Paediatric Cardiology Unit, mimeo, Goldsmiths' College, London.

HOROBIN, G. (1978), The Impossibility of General Practice, paper given at Scottish branch meeting of BSA Medical Sociology Group, Dundee.

ILLICH, I. (1975), 'Medical Nemesis: The Expropriation of Health', Calder and Boyars, London.

JANEWAY, C.A. (1974), Family Medicine - Fad or for Real, 'New England Journal of Medicine', 291, 7, 15 August, pp. 337-43.

JEFFREYS, R. (1974), Natural Rubbish: Deviant Patients in Casualty Departments, paper given at National Deviancy Conference on Medical Ideologies, Bath.

JEWSON, N.D. (1974), Medical Knowledge and the Patronage System in 18th Century England, 'Sociology', 8, 3, pp. 369-85.

JOHNSON, T. (1972), 'Professions and Power', Macmillan, London.

LEY, P. and SPELMAN, M.S. (1967), 'Communication with the Patient', Staples Press, London.

LOFLAND, J. (1976), 'Doing Social Life: The Qualitative Study of Human Interaction in Natural Settings', Wiley, London.

McDONALD, E.B. and PATEL, A.R. (1975), Attitudes Towards Alcoholism, 'British Medical Journal', 2 May, pp.430-1.

MACINTYRE, S. (1976), Who Wants Babies? - The Social Construction of Instincts, in D.L.Barker and S.Allen (eds), 'Sexual Divisions and Society: Process and Change', Tavistock, London, pp.150-73.

MACINTYRE, S. (1977), 'Single and Pregnant', Croom Helm, London.

MECHANIC, D. (1971), The English National Health Service: Some Comparisons with the United States, 'Journal of Health and Social Behaviour', 12, pp.18-29.

NAVARRO, V. (1977), Social Class, Political Power, and the State; their Implications in Medicine, 'International Journal of Health Services', 7, 2, pp.254-92.

PARSONS, T. (1951), 'The Social System', Routledge & Kegan Paul, London.

PHILLIPS, D.L. (1971), 'Knowledge from What - Methods in Social Research', Rand McNally, Chicago.

PILIAVIN, I. and BRIAR, S. (1964), Police Encounters with Juveniles, 'American Journal of Sociology', 69, pp.206-14.

POGGI, G. (1977), The Constitutional State of the 19th Century: An Elementary Conceptual Portrait, 'Sociology', 11, pp.311-32.

ROBINSON, W. (1951), The Logical Structure of Analytical Induction, 'American Sociological Review', 16, pp.812-18.

ROTH, J. (1963), 'Time-Tables - Structuring the Passage of Time in Hospital Treatment and Other Careers', Bobbs-Merrill, Indianapolis.

ROTH, J. (1975), The Treatment of the Sick, in J.Kosa and I.K.Zola (eds), 'Poverty and Health: A Sociological Analysis', Harvard University Press, Cambridge, Mass., pp.214-43.

ROTH, J. (1977), A Yank in the NHS, in A.G.Davis and G.Horobin (eds), 'Medical Encounters', Croom Helm, London, pp.191-205.

SCHEFF, T. (1968), Negotiating Reality: Notes on Power in the Assessment of Responsibility, 'Social Problems', 16, pp.3-17.

SONTAG, S. (1978), 'Illness as Metaphor', Farrar, Strauss and Giroux, New York.

SOROKIN, P. (1956), 'Fads and Foibles in Modern Sociology', Henry Regnery, Chicago.

STIMSON, G. (1977), Social Care and the Role of the General Practitioner, 'Social Science and Medicine', 11, pp.485-90.

STIMSON, G. (1978), Treatment or Control? Dilemmas for Staff in Drug Dependency Clinics, in D.J.West (ed.), 'Problems of Drug Abuse in Britain', University of Cambridge.

STIMSON, G. and WEBB, B. (1975), Going to See the Doctor, Routledge & Kegan Paul, London.

STRONG, P.M. (1977a), Medical Errands, in A.G.Davis and G.Horobin (eds), 'Medical Encounters', Croom Helm, London.

STRONG, P.M. (1977b), Alcoholics, The Sick Role and Bourgeois Medicine, mimeo.

STRONG, P.M. (1979), Sociological Imperialism and the Profession of Medicine: A Critical Examination of the Thesis of Medical Imperialism, 'Social Science and Medicine', 13A, pp.199-215.

STRONG, P.M. (1980), Doctors and Dirty Work: The Case of Alcoholism, 'Sociology of Health and Illness' (forthcoming).

STRONG, P.M. and DAVIS, A.G. (1977), Roles, Role Formats and Medical Encounters: A Cross-cultural Analysis of Staff-Patient Relationships in Children's Clinics, 'Sociological Review', 25, 4, pp.775-800.

STRONG, P.M. and DAVIS, A.G. (1978), Who's Who in Paediatric Encounters: Morality, Expertise and the Generation of Identity and Action in Medical Settings, in A.G.Davis (ed.), 'Relations between Doctors and Patients', Saxon House, London, pp.48-75.

STRONG, P.M. and MAY, D.R. (1980), Sociological Concepts of Childhood, in R.G.Mitchell (ed.), 'Child Health in the Community', second edition, Churchill Livingstone, London (forthcoming).

SUDNOW, D. (1967), 'Passing On: The Social Organization
of Dying', Prentice-Hall, New Jersey.
SUDNOW, D. (1972), Temporal Parameters of Interpersonal
Observation, in D.Sudnow (ed.), 'Studies in Social Inter-
action', Free Press, New York, pp.259-79.
TURNER, R. (1972), Some Formal Properties of Therapy Talk,
in D.Sudnow (ed.), 'Studies in Social Interaction', Free
Press, New York, pp.367-96.
VOYSEY, M. (1975), 'A Constant Burden', Routledge & Kegan
Paul, London.
WAITZKIN, H.K. and WATERMAN, B. (1974), 'The Exploitation
of Illness in Capitalist Society', Bobbs-Merrill, Indian-
apolis.
WEINSTEIN, E. (1966), Towards a Theory of Interpersonal
Tactics, in C.Backman and P.Secord (eds), 'Problems in
Social Psychology', McGraw-Hill, New York, pp.394-8.
WEINSTEIN, E. (1969), The Development of Interpersonal
Competence, in D.Goslin (ed.), 'A Handbook of Sociali-
zation Theory and Research', Rand McNally, Chicago, pp.
753-75.
WEINSTEIN, E. and DEUTSCHBERGER, P. (1964), Tasks,
Bargains and Identities in Social Interaction, 'Social
Forces', 42, 451-6.
WENGLINSKY, M. (1973), Errands, in A.Birenbaum and
E.Sagarin (eds), 'People in Places: The Sociology of the
Familiar', Nelson, London, pp.83-100.
WERTHMAN, C. (1969), Delinquency and Moral Character, in
D.Cressey and D.Ward (eds), 'Delinquency, Crime and Social
Process', Harper and Row, New York, pp.613-22.

Index

Routledge Social Science Series

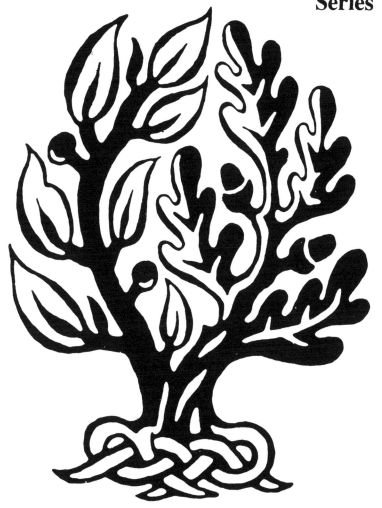

Routledge & Kegan Paul   London, Henley and Boston

39 Store Street, London WC1E 7DD
Broadway House, Newtown Road,
Henley-on-Thames, Oxon RG9 1EN
9 Park Street, Boston, Mass. 02108

Contents

*Authors wishing to submit manuscripts for any series in
this catalogue should send them to the Social Science Editor,
Routledge & Kegan Paul Ltd, 39 Store Street,
London WC1E 7DD*

● *Books so marked are available in paperback
All books are in Metric Demy 8vo format (216 × 138mm approx.)*

International Library of Sociology

General Editor John Rex

GENERAL SOCIOLOGY

Barnsley, J. H. The Social Reality of Ethics. *464 pp.*
Brown, Robert. Explanation in Social Science. *208 pp.*
● Rules and Laws in Sociology. *192 pp.*
Bruford, W. H. Chekhov and His Russia. *A Sociological Study. 244 pp.*
Burton, F. and **Carlen, P.** Official Discourse. *On Discourse Analysis, Government Publications, Ideology. About 140 pp.*
Cain, Maureen E. Society and the Policeman's Role. *326 pp.*
● **Fletcher, Colin.** Beneath the Surface. *An Account of Three Styles of Sociological Research. 221 pp.*
Gibson, Quentin. The Logic of Social Enquiry. *240 pp.*
Glucksmann, M. Structuralist Analysis in Contemporary Social Thought. *212 pp.*
Gurvitch, Georges. Sociology of Law. *Foreword by Roscoe Pound. 264 pp.*
Hinkle, R. Founding Theory of American Sociology 1883-1915. *About 350 pp.*
Homans, George C. Sentiments and Activities. *336 pp.*
Johnson, Harry M. Sociology: *a Systematic Introduction. Foreword by Robert K. Merton. 710 pp.*
● **Keat, Russell** and **Urry, John.** Social Theory as Science. *278 pp.*
Mannheim, Karl. Essays on Sociology and Social Psychology. *Edited by Paul Keckskemeti. With Editorial Note by Adolph Lowe. 344 pp.*
Martindale, Don. The Nature and Types of Sociological Theory. *292 pp.*
● **Maus, Heinz.** A Short History of Sociology. *234 pp.*
Myrdal, Gunnar. Value in Social Theory: *A Collection of Essays on Methodology. Edited by Paul Streeten. 332 pp.*
Ogburn, William F. and **Nimkoff, Meyer F.** A Handbook of Sociology. *Preface by Karl Mannheim. 656 pp. 46 figures. 35 tables.*
Parsons, Talcott, and **Smelser, Neil J.** Economy and Society: *A Study in the Integration of Economic and Social Theory. 362 pp.*
Podgórecki, Adam. Practical Social Sciences. *About 200 pp.*
Raffel, S. Matters of Fact. *A Sociological Inquiry. 152 pp.*
● **Rex, John.** (Ed.) Approaches to Sociology. *Contributions by Peter Abell,* Sociology and the Demystification of the Modern World. *282 pp.*
● **Rex, John** (Ed.) Approaches to Sociology. *Contributions by Peter Abell, Frank Bechhofer, Basil Bernstein, Ronald Fletcher, David Frisby, Miriam Glucksmann, Peter Lassman, Herminio Martins, John Rex, Roland Robertson, John Westergaard and Jock Young. 302 pp.*
Rigby, A. Alternative Realities. *352 pp.*
Roche, M. Phenomenology, Language and the Social Sciences. *374 pp.*
Sahay, A. Sociological Analysis. *220 pp.*

Strasser, Hermann. The Normative Structure of Sociology. *Conservative and Emancipatory Themes in Social Thought. About 340 pp.*
Strong, P. Ceremonial Order of the Clinic. *About 250 pp.*
Urry, John. Reference Groups and the Theory of Revolution. *244 pp.*
Weinberg, E. Development of Sociology in the Soviet Union. *173 pp.*

FOREIGN CLASSICS OF SOCIOLOGY

● **Gerth, H. H.** and **Mills, C. Wright.** From Max Weber: *Essays in Sociology. 502 pp.*
● **Tönnies, Ferdinand.** Community and Association. *(Gemeinschaft and Gesellschaft.) Translated and Supplemented by Charles P. Loomis. Foreword by Pitirim A. Sorokin. 334 pp.*

SOCIAL STRUCTURE

Andreski, Stanislav. Military Organization and Society. *Foreword by Professor A. R. Radcliffe-Brown. 226 pp. 1 folder.*
Carlton, Eric. Ideology and Social Order. *Foreword by Professor Philip Abrahams. About 320 pp.*
Coontz, Sydney H. Population Theories and the Economic Interpretation. *202 pp.*
Coser, Lewis. The Functions of Social Conflict. *204 pp.*
Dickie-Clark, H. F. Marginal Situation: *A Sociological Study of a Coloured Group. 240 pp. 11 tables.*
Giner, S. and **Archer, M. S.** (Eds.). Contemporary Europe. *Social Structures and Cultural Patterns. 336 pp.*
● **Glaser, Barney** and **Strauss, Anselm L.** Status Passage. *A Formal Theory. 212 pp.*
Glass, D. V. (Ed.) Social Mobility in Britain. *Contributions by J. Berent, T. Bottomore, R. C. Chambers, J. Floud, D. V. Glass, J. R. Hall, H. T. Himmelweit, R. K. Kelsall, F. M. Martin, C. A. Moser, R. Mukherjee, and W. Ziegel. 420 pp.*
Kelsall, R. K. Higher Civil Servants in Britain: *From 1870 to the Present Day. 268 pp. 31 tables.*
● **Lawton, Denis.** Social Class, Language and Education. *192 pp.*
McLeish, John. The Theory of Social Change: *Four Views Considered. 128 pp.*
● **Marsh, David C.** The Changing Social Structure of England and Wales, 1871-1961. *Revised edition. 288 pp.*
Menzies, Ken. Talcott Parsons and the Social Image of Man. *About 208 pp.*
● **Mouzelis, Nicos.** Organization and Bureaucracy. *An Analysis of Modern Theories. 240 pp.*
Ossowski, Stanislaw. Class Structure in the Social Consciousness. *210 pp.*
● **Podgórecki, Adam.** Law and Society. *302 pp.*
Renner, Karl. Institutions of Private Law and Their Social Functions. *Edited, with an Introduction and Notes, by O. Kahn-Freud. Translated by Agnes Schwarzschild. 316 pp.*

Rex, J. and **Tomlinson, S.** Colonial Immigrants in a British City. *A Class Analysis. 368 pp.*

Smooha, S. Israel: Pluralism and Conflict. *472 pp.*

Wesolowski, W. Class, Strata and Power. *Trans. and with Introduction by G. Kolankiewicz. 160 pp.*

Zureik, E. Palestinians in Israel. *A Study in Internal Colonialism. 264 pp.*

SOCIOLOGY AND POLITICS

Acton, T. A. Gypsy Politics and Social Change. *316 pp.*

Burton, F. Politics of Legitimacy. *Struggles in a Belfast Community. 250 pp.*

Etzioni-Halevy, E. Political Manipulation and Administrative Power. *A Comparative Study. About 200 pp.*

● **Hechter, Michael.** Internal Colonialism. *The Celtic Fringe in British National Development, 1536–1966. 380 pp.*

Kornhauser, William. The Politics of Mass Society. *272 pp. 20 tables.*

Korpi, W. The Working Class in Welfare Capitalism. *Work, Unions and Politics in Sweden. 472 pp.*

Kroes, R. Soldiers and Students. *A Study of Right- and Left-wing Students. 174 pp.*

Martin, Roderick. Sociology of Power. *About 272 pp.*

Myrdal, Gunnar. The Political Element in the Development of Economic Theory. *Translated from the German by Paul Streeten. 282 pp.*

Wong, S.-L. Sociology and Socialism in Contemporary China. *160 pp.*

Wootton, Graham. Workers, Unions and the State. *188 pp.*

CRIMINOLOGY

Ancel, Marc. Social Defence: *A Modern Approach to Criminal Problems. Foreword by Leon Radzinowicz. 240 pp.*

Athens, L. Violent Criminal Acts and Actors. *About 150 pp.*

Cain, Maureen E. Society and the Policeman's Role. *326 pp.*

Cloward, Richard A. and **Ohlin, Lloyd E.** Delinquency and Opportunity: *A Theory of Delinquent Gangs. 248 pp.*

Downes, David M. The Delinquent Solution. *A Study in Subcultural Theory. 296 pp.*

Friedlander, Kate. The Psycho-Analytical Approach to Juvenile Delinquency: *Theory, Case Studies, Treatment. 320 pp.*

Gleuck, Sheldon and **Eleanor.** Family Environment and Delinquency. *With the statistical assistance of Rose W. Kneznek. 340 pp.*

Lopez-Rey, Manuel. Crime. *An Analytical Appraisal. 288 pp.*

Mannheim, Hermann. Comparative Criminology: *a Text Book. Two volumes. 442 pp. and 380 pp.*

Morris, Terence. The Criminal Area: *A Study in Social Ecology. Foreword by Hermann Mannheim. 232 pp. 25 tables. 4 maps.*

Podgorecki, A. and **Łos, M.** *Multidimensional Sociology. About 380 pp.*

Rock, Paul. Making People Pay. *338 pp.*

● **Taylor, Ian, Walton, Paul,** and **Young, Jock.** The New Criminology. *For a Social Theory of Deviance. 325 pp.*

● **Taylor, Ian, Walton, Paul** and **Young, Jock.** (Eds) Critical Criminology. *268 pp.*

SOCIAL PSYCHOLOGY

Bagley, Christopher. The Social Psychology of the Epileptic Child. *320 pp.*

Brittan, Arthur. Meanings and Situations. *224 pp.*

Carroll, J. Break-Out from the Crystal Palace. *200 pp.*

● **Fleming, C. M.** Adolescence: Its Social Psychology. *With an Introduction to recent findings from the fields of Anthropology, Physiology, Medicine, Psychometrics and Sociometry. 288 pp.*

● The Social Psychology of Education: *An Introduction and Guide to Its Study. 136 pp.*

Linton, Ralph. The Cultural Background of Personality. *132 pp.*

● **Mayo, Elton.** The Social Problems of an Industrial Civilization. *With an Appendix on the Political Problem. 180 pp.*

Ottaway, A. K. C. Learning Through Group Experience. *176 pp.*

Plummer, Ken. Sexual Stigma. *An Interactionist Account. 254 pp.*

● **Rose, Arnold M.** (Ed.) Human Behaviour and Social Processes: *an Interactionist Approach. Contributions by Arnold M. Rose, Ralph H. Turner, Anselm Strauss, Everett C. Hughes, E. Franklin Frazier, Howard S. Becker et al. 696 pp.*

Smelser, Neil J. Theory of Collective Behaviour. *448 pp.*

Stephenson, Geoffrey M. The Development of Conscience. *128 pp.*

Young, Kimball. Handbook of Social Psychology. *658 pp. 16 figures. 10 tables.*

SOCIOLOGY OF THE FAMILY

Bell, Colin R. Middle Class Families: *Social and Geographical Mobility. 224 pp.*

Burton, Lindy. Vulnerable Children. *272 pp.*

Gavron, Hannah. The Captive Wife: *Conflicts of Household Mothers. 190 pp.*

George, Victor and **Wilding, Paul.** Motherless Families. *248 pp.*

Klein, Josephine. Samples from English Cultures.

    1. Three Preliminary Studies and Aspects of Adult Life in England. *447 pp.*

    2. Child-Rearing Practices and Index. *247 pp.*

Klein, Viola. The Feminine Character. *History of an Ideology. 244 pp.*

McWhinnie, Alexina M. Adopted Children. *How They Grow Up. 304 pp.*

● **Morgan, D. H. J.** Social Theory and the Family. *About 320 pp.*

● **Myrdal, Alva** and **Klein, Viola.** Women's Two Roles: *Home and Work. 238 pp. 27 tables.*

Parsons, Talcott and **Bales, Robert F.** Family: Socialization and Interaction Process. *In collaboration with James Olds, Morris Zelditch and Philip E. Slater. 456 pp. 50 figures and tables.*

SOCIAL SERVICES

Bastide, Roger. The Sociology of Mental Disorder. *Translated from the French by Jean McNeil. 260 pp.*

Carlebach, Julius. Caring For Children in Trouble. *266 pp.*

George, Victor. Foster Care. *Theory and Practice. 234 pp.*
Social Security: *Beveridge and After. 258 pp.*

George, V. and **Wilding, P.** Motherless Families. *248 pp.*

● **Goetschius, George W.** Working with Community Groups. *256 pp.*

Goetschius, George W. and **Tash, Joan.** Working with Unattached Youth. *416 pp.*

Heywood, Jean S. Children in Care. *The Development of the Service for the Deprived Child. Third revised edition. 284 pp.*

King, Roy D., Ranes, Norma V. and **Tizard, Jack.** Patterns of Residential Care. *356 pp.*

Leigh, John. Young People and Leisure. *256 pp.*

● **Mays, John.** (Ed.) Penelope Hall's Social Services of England and Wales. *About 324 pp.*

Morris, Mary. Voluntary Work and the Welfare State. *300 pp.*

Nokes, P. L. The Professional Task in Welfare Practice. *152 pp.*

Timms, Noel. Psychiatric Social Work in Great Britain (1939-1962). *280 pp.*

● Social Casework: *Principles and Practice. 256 pp.*

SOCIOLOGY OF EDUCATION

Banks, Olive. Parity and Prestige in English Secondary Education: a Study in Educational Sociology. *272 pp.*

● **Blyth, W. A. L.** English Primary Education. *A Sociological Description.* 2. Background. *168 pp.*

Collier, K. G. The Social Purposes of Education: *Personal and Social Values in Education. 268 pp.*

Evans, K. M. Sociometry and Education. *158 pp.*

● **Ford, Julienne.** Social Class and the Comprehensive School. *192 pp.*

Foster, P. J. Education and Social Change in Ghana. *336 pp. 3 maps.*

Fraser, W. R. Education and Society in Modern France. *150 pp.*

Grace, Gerald R. Role Conflict and the Teacher. *150 pp.*

Hans, Nicholas. New Trends in Education in the Eighteenth Century. *278 pp. 19 tables.*

● Comparative Education: *A Study of Educational Factors and Traditions. 360 pp.*

● **Hargreaves, David.** Interpersonal Relations and Education. *432 pp.*

● Social Relations in a Secondary School. *240 pp.*
School Organization and Pupil Involvement. *A Study of Secondary Schools.*

- **Mannheim, Karl** and **Stewart, W.A.C.** An Introduction to the Sociology of Education. *206 pp.*
- **Musgrove, F.** Youth and the Social Order. *176 pp.*
- **Ottaway, A. K. C.** Education and Society: An Introduction to the Sociology of Education. *With an Introduction by W. O. Lester Smith. 212 pp.*
  Peers, Robert. Adult Education: *A Comparative Study. Revised edition. 398 pp.*
  Stratta, Erica. The Education of Borstal Boys. *A Study of their Educational Experiences prior to, and during, Borstal Training. 256 pp.*
- **Taylor, P. H., Reid, W. A.** and **Holley, B. J.** The English Sixth Form. *A Case Study in Curriculum Research. 198 pp.*

SOCIOLOGY OF CULTURE

Eppel, E. M. and **M.** Adolescents and Morality: *A Study of some Moral Values and Dilemmas of Working Adolescents in the Context of a changing Climate of Opinion. Foreword by W. J. H. Sprott. 268 pp. 39 tables.*
- **Fromm, Erich.** The Fear of Freedom. *286 pp.*
-     The Sane Society. *400 pp.*
  Johnson, L. The Cultural Critics. *From Matthew Arnold to Raymond Williams. 233 pp.*
  Mannheim, Karl. Essays on the Sociology of Culture. *Edited by Ernst Mannheim in co-operation with Paul Kecskemeti. Editorial Note by Adolph Lowe. 280 pp.*
  Zijderfeld, A. C. On Clichés. *The Supersedure of Meaning by Function in Modernity. About 132 pp.*

SOCIOLOGY OF RELIGION

Argyle, Michael and **Beit-Hallahmi, Benjamin.** The Social Psychology of Religion. *About 256 pp.*
Glasner, Peter E. The Sociology of Secularisation. *A Critique of a Concept. About 180 pp.*
Hall, J. R. The Ways Out. *Utopian Communal Groups in an Age of Babylon. 280 pp.*
Ranson, S., Hinings, B. and **Bryman, A.** Clergy, Ministers and Priests. *216 pp.*
Stark, Werner. The Sociology of Religion. *A Study of Christendom.*
   Volume II. *Sectarian Religion. 368 pp.*
   Volume III. *The Universal Church. 464 pp.*
   Volume IV. *Types of Religious Man. 352 pp.*
   Volume V. *Types of Religious Culture. 464 pp.*
Turner, B. S. Weber and Islam. *216 pp.*
Watt, W. Montgomery. Islam and the Integration of Society. *320 pp.*

SOCIOLOGY OF ART AND LITERATURE

Jarvie, Ian C. Towards a Sociology of the Cinema. *A Comparative Essay on the Structure and Functioning of a Major Entertainment Industry. 405 pp.*

Rust, Frances S. Dance in Society. *An Analysis of the Relationships between the Social Dance and Society in England from the Middle Ages to the Present Day. 256 pp. 8 pp. of plates.*

Schücking, L. L. The Sociology of Literary Taste. *112 pp.*

Wolff, Janet. Hermeneutic Philosophy and the Sociology of Art. *150 pp.*

SOCIOLOGY OF KNOWLEDGE

Diesing, P. Patterns of Discovery in the Social Sciences. *262 pp.*

● **Douglas, J. D.** (Ed.) Understanding Everyday Life. *370 pp.*

Glasner, B. Essential Interactionism. *About 220 pp.*

● **Hamilton, P.** Knowledge and Social Structure. *174 pp.*

Jarvie, I. C. Concepts and Society. *232 pp.*

Mannheim, Karl. Essays on the Sociology of Knowledge. *Edited by Paul Kecskemeti. Editorial Note by Adolph Lowe. 353 pp.*

Remmling, Gunter W. The Sociology of Karl Mannheim. *With a Bibliographical Guide to the Sociology of Knowledge, Ideological Analysis, and Social Planning. 255 pp.*

Remmling, Gunter W. (Ed.) Towards the Sociology of Knowledge. *Origin and Development of a Sociological Thought Style. 463 pp.*

URBAN SOCIOLOGY

Aldridge, M. The British New Towns. *A Programme Without a Policy. About 250 pp.*

Ashworth, William. The Genesis of Modern British Town Planning: *A Study in Economic and Social History of the Nineteenth and Twentieth Centuries. 288 pp.*

Brittan, A. The Privatised World. *196 pp.*

Cullingworth, J. B. Housing Needs and Planning Policy: *A Restatement of the Problems of Housing Need and 'Overspill' in England and Wales. 232 pp. 44 tables. 8 maps.*

Dickinson, Robert E. City and Region: *A Geographical Interpretation. 608 pp. 125 figures.*

The West European City: *A Geographical Interpretation. 600 pp. 129 maps. 29 plates.*

Humphreys, Alexander J. New Dubliners: *Urbanization and the Irish Family. Foreword by George C. Homans. 304 pp.*

Jackson, Brian. Working Class Community: *Some General Notions raised by a Series of Studies in Northern England. 192 pp.*

● **Mann, P. H.** An Approach to Urban Sociology. *240 pp.*

Mellor, J. R. Urban Sociology in an Urbanized Society. *326 pp.*

Morris, R. N. and **Mogey, J.** The Sociology of Housing. *Studies at Berinsfield. 232 pp. 4 pp. plates.*

9

Rosser, C. and **Harris, C.** The Family and Social Change. *A Study of Family and Kinship in a South Wales Town. 352 pp. 8 maps.*

● **Stacey, Margaret, Batsone, Eric, Bell, Colin** and **Thurcott, Anne.** Power, Persistence and Change. *A Second Study of Banbury. 196 pp.*

RURAL SOCIOLOGY

Mayer, Adrian C. Peasants in the Pacific. *A Study of Fiji Indian Rural Society. 248 pp. 20 plates.*

Williams, W. M. The Sociology of an English Village: *Gosforth. 272 pp. 12 figures. 13 tables.*

SOCIOLOGY OF INDUSTRY AND DISTRIBUTION

Dunkerley, David. The Foreman. *Aspects of Task and Structure. 192 pp.*

Eldridge, J. E. T. Industrial Disputes. *Essays in the Sociology of Industrial Relations. 288 pp.*

Hollowell, Peter G. The Lorry Driver. *272 pp.*

● **Oxaal, I., Barnett, T.** and **Booth, D.** (Eds) Beyond the Sociology of Development. *Economy and Society in Latin America and Africa. 295 pp.*

Smelser, Neil J. Social Change in the Industrial Revolution: *An Application of Theory to the Lancashire Cotton Industry, 1770–1840. 468 pp. 12 figures. 14 tables.*

Watson, T. J. The Personnel Managers. *A Study in the Sociology of Work and Employment. 262 pp.*

ANTHROPOLOGY

Brandel-Syrier, Mia. Reeftown Elite. *A Study of Social Mobility in a Modern African Community on the Reef. 376 pp.*

Dickie-Clark, H. F. The Marginal Situation. *A Sociological Study of a Coloured Group. 236 pp.*

Dube, S. C. Indian Village. *Foreword by Morris Edward Opler. 276 pp. 4 plates.*

India's Changing Villages: *Human Factors in Community Development. 260 pp. 8 plates. 1 map.*

Firth, Raymond. Malay Fishermen. *Their Peasant Economy. 420 pp. 17 pp. plates.*

Gulliver, P. H. Social Control in an African Society: a Study of the Arusha, Agricultural Masai of Northern Tanganyika. *320 pp. 8 plates. 10 figures.*

Family Herds. *288 pp.*

Jarvie, Ian C. The Revolution in Anthropology. *268 pp.*

Little, Kenneth L. Mende of Sierra Leone. *308 pp. and folder.*

Negroes in Britain. *With a New Introduction and Contemporary Study by Leonard Bloom. 320 pp.*

Madan, G. R. Western Sociologists on Indian Society. *Marx, Spencer, Weber, Durkheim, Pareto. 384 pp.*

Mayer, A. C. Peasants in the Pacific. *A Study of Fiji Indian Rural Society. 248 pp.*

Meer, Fatima. Race and Suicide in South Africa. *325 pp.*

Smith, Raymond T. The Negro Family in British Guiana: *Family Structure and Social Status in the Villages. With a Foreword by Meyer Fortes. 314 pp. 8 plates. 1 figure. 4 maps.*

SOCIOLOGY AND PHILOSOPHY

Barnsley, John H. The Social Reality of Ethics. *A Comparative Analysis of Moral Codes. 448 pp.*

Diesing, Paul. Patterns of Discovery in the Social Sciences. *362 pp.*

● **Douglas, Jack D.** (Ed.) Understanding Everyday Life. *Toward the Reconstruction of Sociological Knowledge. Contributions by Alan F. Blum, Aaron W. Cicourel, Norman K. Denzin, Jack D. Douglas, John Heeren, Peter McHugh, Peter K. Manning, Melvin Power, Matthew Speier, Roy Turner, D. Lawrence Wieder, Thomas P. Wilson and Don H. Zimmerman. 370 pp.*

Gorman, Robert A. The Dual Vision. *Alfred Schutz and the Myth of Phenomenological Social Science. About 300 pp.*

Jarvie, Ian C. Concepts and Society. *216 pp.*

Kilminster, R. Praxis and Method. *A Sociological Dialogue with Lukács, Gramsci and the early Frankfurt School. About 304 pp.*

● **Pelz, Werner.** The Scope of Understanding in Sociology. *Towards a More Radical Reorientation in the Social Humanistic Sciences. 283 pp.*

Roche, Maurice. Phenomenology, Language and the Social Sciences. *371 pp.*

Sahay, Arun. Sociological Analysis. *212 pp.*

Slater, P. Origin and Significance of the Frankfurt School. *A Marxist Perspective. About 192 pp.*

Spurling, L. Phenomenology and the Social World. *The Philosophy of Merleau-Ponty and its Relation to the Social Sciences. 222 pp.*

Wilson, H. T. The American Ideology. *Science, Technology and Organization as Modes of Rationality. 368 pp.*

International Library of Anthropology

General Editor   Adam Kuper

Ahmed, A. S. Millenium and Charisma Among Pathans. *A Critical Essay in Social Anthropology. 192 pp.*
Pukhtun Economy and Society. *About 360 pp.*

Brown, Paula. The Chimbu. *A Study of Change in the New Guinea Highlands. 151 pp.*

Foner, N. Jamaica Farewell. *200 pp.*

Gudeman, Stephen. Relationships, Residence and the Individual. *A Rural Panamanian Community. 288 pp. 11 plates, 5 figures, 2 maps, 10 tables.*

The Demise of a Rural Economy. *From Subsistence to Capitalism in a Latin American Village. 160 pp.*

Hamnett, Ian. Chieftainship and Legitimacy. *An Anthropological Study of Executive Law in Lesotho. 163 pp.*

Hanson, F. Allan. Meaning in Culture. *127 pp.*

Humphreys, S. C. Anthropology and the Greeks. *288 pp.*

Karp, I. Fields of Change Among the Iteso of Kenya. *140 pp.*

Lloyd, P. C. Power and Independence. *Urban Africans' Perception of Social Inequality. 264 pp.*

Parry, J. P. Caste and Kinship in Kangra. *352 pp. Illustrated.*

Pettigrew, Joyce. Robber Noblemen. *A Study of the Political System of the Sikh Jats. 284 pp.*

Street, Brian V. The Savage in Literature. *Representations of 'Primitive' Society in English Fiction, 1858–1920. 207 pp.*

Van Den Berghe, Pierre L. Power and Privilege at an African University. *278 pp.*

International Library of Social Policy

General Editor Kathleen Jones

Bayley, M. Mental Handicap and Community Care. *426 pp.*

Bottoms, A. E. and **McClean, J. D.** Defendants in the Criminal Process. *284 pp.*

Butler, J. R. Family Doctors and Public Policy. *208 pp.*

Davies, Martin. Prisoners of Society. *Attitudes and Aftercare. 204 pp.*

Gittus, Elizabeth. Flats, Families and the Under-Fives. *285 pp.*

Holman, Robert. Trading in Children. *A Study of Private Fostering. 355 pp.*

Jeffs, A. Young People and the Youth Service. *About 180 pp.*

Jones, Howard, and **Cornes, Paul.** Open Prisons. *288 pp.*

Jones, Kathleen. History of the Mental Health Service. *428 pp.*

Jones, Kathleen, with **Brown, John, Cunningham, W. J., Roberts, Julian** and **Williams, Peter.** Opening the Door. *A Study of New Policies for the Mentally Handicapped. 278 pp.*

Karn, Valerie. Retiring to the Seaside. *About 280 pp. 2 maps. Numerous tables.*

King, R. D. and **Elliot, K. W.** Albany: Birth of a Prison—End of an Era. *394 pp.*

Thomas, J. E. The English Prison Officer since 1850: *A Study in Conflict. 258 pp.*

Walton, R. G. Women in Social Work. *303 pp.*

● **Woodward, J.** To Do the Sick No Harm. *A Study of the British Voluntary Hospital System to 1875. 234 pp.*

International Library of Welfare and Philosophy

General Editors Noel Timms and David Watson

● **McDermott, F. E.** (Ed.) Self-Determination in Social Work. *A Collection of Essays on Self-determination and Related Concepts by Philosophers and Social Work Theorists. Contributors: F. B. Biestek, S. Bernstein, A. Keith-Lucas, D. Sayer, H. H. Perelman, C. Whittington, R. F. Stalley, F. E. McDermott, I. Berlin, H. J. McCloskey, H. L. A. Hart, J. Wilson, A. I. Melden, S. I. Benn. 254 pp.*

● **Plant, Raymond.** Community and Ideology. *104 pp.*

Ragg, Nicholas M. People Not Cases. *A Philosophical Approach to Social Work. About 250 pp.*

● **Timms, Noel** and **Watson, David.** (Eds) Talking About Welfare. *Readings in Philosophy and Social Policy. Contributors: T. H. Marshall, R. B. Brandt, G. H. von Wright, K. Nielsen, M. Cranston, R. M. Titmuss, R. S. Downie, E. Telfer, D. Donnison, J. Benson, P. Leonard, A. Keith-Lucas, D. Walsh, I. T. Ramsey. 320 pp.*

● (Eds). Philosophy in Social Work. *250 pp.*

● **Weale, A.** Equality and Social Policy. *164 pp.*

Primary Socialization, Language and Education

General Editor Basil Bernstein

Adlam, Diana S., *with the assistance of Geoffrey Turner and Lesley Lineker.* Code in Context. *About 272 pp.*

Bernstein, Basil. Class, Codes and Control. *3 volumes.*

● 1. *Theoretical Studies Towards a Sociology of Language. 254 pp.*

2. *Applied Studies Towards a Sociology of Language. 377 pp.*

● 3. *Towards a Theory of Educational Transmission. 167 pp.*

Brandis, W. and **Bernstein, B.** Selection and Control. *176 pp.*

Brandis, Walter and **Henderson, Dorothy.** Social Class, Language and Communication. *288 pp.*

Cook-Gumperz, Jenny. Social Control and Socialization. *A Study of Class Differences in the Language of Maternal Control. 290 pp.*

● **Gahagan, D. M** and **G. A.** Talk Reform. *Exploration in Language for Infant School Children. 160 pp.*

Hawkins, P. R. Social Class, the Nominal Group and Verbal Strategies. *About 220 pp.*

Robinson, W. P. and **Rackstraw, Susan D. A.** A Question of Answers. *2 volumes. 192 pp. and 180 pp.*

Turner, Geoffrey J. and **Mohan, Bernard A.** A Linguistic Description and Computer Programme for Children's Speech. *208 pp.*

Reports of the Institute of Community Studies

Baker, J. The Neighbourhood Advice Centre. A Community Project in Camden. *320 pp.*

● **Cartwright, Ann.** Patients and their Doctors. *A Study of General Practice. 304 pp.*

Dench, Geoff. Maltese in London. *A Case-study in the Erosion of Ethnic Consciousness. 302 pp.*

Jackson, Brian and **Marsden, Dennis.** Education and the Working Class: *Some General Themes raised by a Study of 88 Working-class Children in a Northern Industrial City. 268 pp. 2 folders.*

Marris, Peter. The Experience of Higher Education. *232 pp. 27 tables.*

● Loss and Change. *192 pp.*

Marris, Peter and **Rein, Martin.** Dilemmas of Social Reform. *Poverty and Community Action in the United States. 256 pp.*

Marris, Peter and **Somerset, Anthony.** African Businessmen. *A Study of Entrepreneurship and Development in Keyna. 256 pp.*

Mills, Richard. Young Outsiders: *a Study in Alternative Communities. 216 pp.*

Runciman, W. G. Relative Deprivation and Social Justice. *A Study of Attitudes to Social Inequality in Twentieth-Century England. 352 pp.*

Willmott, Peter. Adolescent Boys in East London. *230 pp.*

Willmott, Peter and **Young, Michael.** Family and Class in a London Suburb. *202 pp. 47 tables.*

Young, Michael and **McGeeney, Patrick.** Learning Begins at Home. *A Study of a Junior School and its Parents. 128 pp.*

Young, Michael and **Willmott, Peter.** Family and Kinship in East London. *Foreword by Richard M. Titmuss. 252 pp. 39 tables.*

The Symmetrical Family. *410 pp.*

Reports of the Institute for Social Studies in Medical Care

Cartwright, Ann, Hockey, Lisbeth and **Anderson, John J.** Life Before Death. *310 pp.*

Dunnell, Karen and **Cartwright, Ann.** Medicine Takers, Prescribers and Hoarders. *190 pp.*

Farrell, C. My Mother Said. . . . *A Study of the Way Young People Learned About Sex and Birth Control. 200 pp.*

Medicine, Illness and Society

General Editor W. M. Williams

Hall, David J. Social Relations & Innovation. *Changing the State of Play in Hospitals. 232 pp.*

Hall, David J., and **Stacey, M.** (Eds) Beyond Separation. *234 pp.*

Robinson, David. The Process of Becoming Ill. *142 pp.*

Stacey, Margaret *et al.* Hospitals, Children and Their Families. *The Report of a Pilot Study. 202 pp.*

Stimson G. V. and **Webb, B.** Going to See the Doctor. *The Consultation Process in General Practice. 155 pp.*

Monographs in Social Theory

General Editor Arthur Brittan

● **Barnes, B.** Scientific Knowledge and Sociological Theory. *192 pp.*

Bauman, Zygmunt. Culture as Praxis. *204 pp.*

● **Dixon, Keith.** Sociological Theory. *Pretence and Possibility. 142 pp.*

Meltzer, B. N., Petras, J. W. and **Reynolds, L. T.** Symbolic Interactionism. *Genesis, Varieties and Criticisms. 144 pp.*

● **Smith, Anthony D.** The Concept of Social Change. *A Critique of the Functionalist Theory of Social Change. 208 pp.*

Routledge Social Science Journals

The British Journal of Sociology. *Editor – Angus Stewart; Associate Editor – Leslie Sklair. Vol. 1, No. 1 – March 1950 and Quarterly. Roy. 8vo. All back issues available. An international journal publishing original papers in the field of sociology and related areas.*

15

Community Work. *Edited by David Jones and Marjorie Mayo. 1973. Published annually.*

Economy and Society. *Vol. 1, No. 1. February 1972 and Quarterly. Metric Roy. 8vo. A journal for all social scientists covering sociology, philosophy, anthropology, economics and history. All back numbers available.*

Ethnic and Racial Studies. *Editor – John Stone. Vol. 1 – 1978. Published quarterly.*

Religion. Journal of Religion and Religions. *Chairman of Editorial Board, Ninian Smart. Vol. 1, No. 1, Spring 1971. A journal with an inter-disciplinary approach to the study of the phenomena of religion. All back numbers available.*

Sociology of Health and Illness. *A Journal of Medical Sociology. Editor – Alan Davies; Associate Editor – Ray Jobling. Vol. 1, Spring 1979. Published 3 times per annum.*

Year Book of Social Policy in Britain, The. *Edited by Kathleen Jones. 1971. Published annually.*

Social and Psychological Aspects of Medical Practice

Editor Trevor Silverstone

Lader, Malcolm. Psychophysiology of Mental Illness. *280 pp.*
● **Silverstone, Trevor** and **Turner, Paul.** Drug Treatment in Psychiatry. *Revised edition. 256 pp.*
Whiteley, J. S. and **Gordon, J.** Group Approaches in Psychiatry. *256 pp.*

Printed and bound by CPI Group (UK) Ltd, Croydon, CR0 4YY

22/10/2024

01777620-0001